Sports Massage

Hands-On Guides for Therapists

Susan Findlay, BSc

North London School of Sports Massage

Human Kinetics

Library of Congress Cataloging-in-Publication Data

Findlay, Susan, 1956-
  Sports massage / Susan Findlay.
     p. ; cm. -- (Hands-on guides for therapists)
  ISBN-13: 978-0-7360-8260-0 (soft cover)
  ISBN-10: 0-7360-8260-3 (soft cover)
1. Sports massage. I. Title. II. Series: Hands-on guides for therapists.
  [DNLM: 1. Massage--methods. 2. Programmed Instruction. 3. Sports Medicine. WB 18.2
F494s 2010]
  RC1226.F56 2010
  615.8'22088796--dc22

                          2009032812

ISBN-10: 0-7360-8260-3 (print)
ISBN-13: 978-0-7360-8260-0 (print)

Copyright © 2010 by Susan Findlay

Acquisitions Editor: John Dickinson, PhD; **Developmental Editor:** Amanda S. Ewing; **Assistant Editors:** Casey A. Gentis and Melissa J. Zavala; **Copyeditor:** Patsy Fortney; **Permission Manager:** Dalene Reeder; **Graphic Designer:** Nancy Rasmus; **Graphic Artist:** Yvonne Griffith; **Cover Designer:** Bob Reuther; **Photographer (cover):** Nigel Farrow; **Photographer (interior):** Nigel Farrow; **Visual Production Assistant:** Joyce Brumfield; **Photo Production Manager:** Jason Allen; **Art Manager:** Kelly Hendren; **Associate Art Manager:** Alan L. Wilborn; **Illustrator:** Jason M. McAlexander, MFA; **Printer:** United Graphics

We thank the North London School of Sports Massage in London, England, for assistance in providing the location for the photo shoot for this book.

Printed in the United States of America   10 9 8 7 6 5 4 3 2

The paper in this book is certified under a sustainable forestry program.

Human Kinetics
Web site: www.HumanKinetics.com

United States: Human Kinetics
P.O. Box 5076
Champaign, IL 61825-5076
800-747-4457
e-mail: humank@hkusa.com

Canada: Human Kinetics
475 Devonshire Road Unit 100
Windsor, ON N8Y 2L5
800-465-7301 (in Canada only)
e-mail: info@hkcanada.com

Europe: Human Kinetics
107 Bradford Road
Stanningley
Leeds LS28 6AT, United Kingdom
+44 (0) 113 255 5665
e-mail: hk@hkeurope.com

Australia: Human Kinetics
57A Price Avenue
Lower Mitcham, South Australia 5062
08 8372 0999
e-mail: info@hkaustralia.com

New Zealand: Human Kinetics
P.O. Box 80
Torrens Park, South Australia 5062
0800 222 062
e-mail: info@hknewzealand.com

Contents

7 Sports Massage for Supine Positions 86

8 Sports Massage for Side-Lying Positions 102

PART IV   Sports Massage Programmes and Management

9 Client Assessment 114

10 Event Massage 141

11 Special Populations 151

Series Preface

Massage may be one of the oldest therapies still used today. At present more therapists than ever before are practicing an ever-expanding range of massage techniques. Many of these techniques are taught through massage schools and within degree courses. Our need now is to provide the best clinical and educational resources that will enable massage therapists to learn the required techniques for delivering massage therapy to clients. Human Kinetics has developed the Hands-On Guides for Therapists series with this in mind.

The Hands-On Guides for Therapists series provides specific tools of assessment and treatment that fall well within the realm of massage therapists but may also be useful for other bodyworkers, such as osteopaths and fitness instructors. Each book in the series is a step-by-step guide to delivering the techniques to clients. Each book features a full-colour interior packed with photos illustrating every technique. Tips provide handy advice to help you adjust your technique, and the Client Talk boxes contain examples of how the techniques can be used with clients who have particular problems. Throughout each book are questions that enable you to test your knowledge and skill, which will be particularly helpful if you are attempting to pass a qualification exam. We've even provided the answers too!

You might be using a book from the Hands-On Guides for Therapists series to obtain the required skills to help you pass a course or to brush up on skills you learned in the past. You might be a course tutor looking for ways to make massage therapy come alive with your students. This series provides easy-to-follow steps that will make the transition from theory to practice seem effortless. The Hands-On Guides for Therapists series is an essential resource for all those who are serious about massage therapy.

Preface

When asked to write this book, I was faced with the difficult task of determining the definition of sports massage within the industry. Is sports massage defined by the techniques we use and the manner in which we use them, or does the definition simply depend on the clients we work with? The answer is not clear cut because it varies not only from country to country but also from person to person.

Massage originated in ancient civilizations. In its simplest form, people would instinctively rub or hold an injured area in order to relieve pain. Massage has evolved into many forms, but the original elements are still evident in all types. Today a common definition has emerged from the name itself, *sports massage*, which is the application of a variety of soft tissue techniques to maximize the performance of athletes. This is partially true, but the manner in which we get our results will often include remedial techniques such as soft tissue release or muscle energy techniques. Furthermore, it can also be argued that the same techniques used in sports massage are not exclusive for athletes; rather, they can be applied to those who do not participate in any sport or have just a passing interest in physical activity. This is why there is such a wide variety of definitions of sports massage.

Whomever you are working with, massage has a holistic result despite the varying opinions about a lack of evidenced-based research on massage. It can be difficult to quantify data when conducting any research because there are so many variables to consider: the therapist, the client, the training, the style, and the techniques. Yet from my years of experience, I've seen how effective massage therapy can be, which is all the evidence I've needed to continue doing the job.

This book provides sports massage therapists with the essential tools for delivering a well-thought-out massage session in a sport or general context. Part I covers how to get started and what you need to consider before you start. It specifies when you should and should not use massage and the benefits that can be derived from hands-on therapy, and it features a quick-reference pathology section that will be useful throughout your career. Parts II and III focus on the application of the techniques by demonstrating multiple positions, which will allow you to form your own style. Part IV takes you through the assessment process using a variety of tools, beginning with a verbal consultation, moving on to visual assessments, and ending with movement and strength testing. Charts and questionnaires will help you design your own consultation forms, or you can use the ones provided. The final chapters cover working in a sporting environment, whether at a local event or in an elite setting.

eBook
available at
HumanKinetics.com

You will find talk boxes and tips throughout each chapter. Talk boxes focus on experiential information and give practical advice. Tips draw out important points to remember or summarize large sections for easy reference. You can refer to both as needed to reinforce your learning.

Sports Massage emphasizes working efficiently and applying techniques with ease and sensitivity. This approach will make your job easier, increase your longevity as a therapist, and improve the quality of your touch. You will be able to address and correct the common injuries that therapists often incur as a result of incorrect positioning and movement. You will also be able to apply the specialized techniques in a more effective and controlled manner.

Your training as a sports massage therapist should not stop here; rather, it should evolve through the addition of remedial and advanced techniques. With a good foundation, you will have greater success in all areas.

Acknowledgments

This book was written and supported by the efforts of many people, all of whom I want to give my heartfelt thanks to.

A special thanks to Chris Salvary who spent the Christmas holiday proof reading my material. To Albie McMahon for his initial support and editing. To Elizabeth Soames who took the time out of her busy schedule to write a piece about working with an elite sports team.

My thanks and appreciation to John Dickinson and Amanda Ewing from Human Kinetics who gave unending advice and support. To Jane Johnson, whose idea for this series originated with.

I have had the privilege of working with a great team of teachers that have supported me throughout this venture, a family that has kept me laughing and focused, and friends who have remained friends despite my lack of participation in their lives while I wrote this book.

I thank all of you that are true to the profession and only want the best for the future, you are the future.

PART I

Getting Started With Sports Massage

In chapters 1 through 3 you will find relevant information about how to get started as a sports massage therapist. Chapters 1 and 2 cover your foundational techniques, the appropriate use of those techniques within a session, and the benefits and contraindications associated with them. Chapter 2 contains a section on general pathology that will help further develop your abilities as a safe and effective therapist. This section will enable you to work more holistically and make important decisions about what modifications are needed in order to accommodate the body's current state of health.

The pathology section serves as a quick reference guide to various systemic or soft tissue conditions and details the massage modifications necessary to deliver an effective and safe soft tissue treatment. Chapter 2 warrants revisiting over the course of time as and when it is needed. Chapter 3 helps you make decisions about where you are likely to offer your services as well as the practical information needed in order to set up.

At the end of each chapter are Quick Questions that reinforce the material covered and help you to focus on the main points.

Introduction to Sports Massage

Welcome to sports massage. If you are new to this form of massage or have never had any formal training, or if you want to improve your skills and understanding of sports massage, then this is the place to start. Whatever stage you are at in your practice, you will find useful tips about how to start out or improve your practice throughout this book. This chapter takes you to the beginning of the story, laying the foundation about how sports massage works, when and where you can use it, and the scope of possibilities it can offer a client.

What Is Sports Massage?

Sports massage is a deep form of soft tissue work that is applied in a sporting context. It consists of a variety of techniques that include effleurage, petrissage, tapotement, vibration, compression, deep strokes and friction. Some of the more advanced techniques range from soft tissue release, neuromuscular techniques, myofascial release, muscle energy techniques, positional release, connective tissue manipulation and many more. The main focus of sports massage is to help the athlete achieve peak performance and remain injury free as well as to support the healing of injuries. As a sports massage therapist, you should be able to perform an appropriate range of assessment and evaluation processes as well as recognise common sports injuries. You should also be able to design and implement comprehensive treatment plans with realistic and achievable goals.

Who Should Be Treated?

Sports massage is not limited to athletes. It is appropriate for anyone who is in need of remedial or soft tissue work irrespective of age, level of fitness or gender. The remedial effects of sports massage can be beneficial in the postsurgical setting; as an adjunct to physiotherapy, osteopathy or chiropractic in rehabilitative therapy; or as a health benefit within the office environment. Although the name might imply a sporting clientele, it is a therapy appropriate to all.

Within the sporting context, experts recommend that athletes use sports massage as a regular part of their training programs rather than having sporadic massage sessions. Because regular massage has cumulative benefits, it is more effective as a performance enhancement than occasional massage, which could disrupt performance. Athletes new to massage should not have their first sports massage sessions close to an upcoming event; they are better served by starting with regular sessions after an event.

How Does Sports Massage Work?

Up until now, research has not been able to quantify how and why massage works. Although it is offered widely within the fitness industry and medical fields, evidenced-based research has not so far provided satisfactory answers about the mechanisms and benefits of massage. The studies that have been done are confusing and give conflicting or, at best, equivocal results. Until more high-quality, methodologically sound studies are conducted, the best method of determining the benefits of massage is to gauge the response of the athlete.

It is believed that sports massage works both mechanically and reflexively. Mechanically, massage works with the skin, fascia, muscle and connective tissues through pressure and movement. It softens, lengthens or stretches the soft tissue, thereby increasing the range of motion within soft tissue structures, which can lead to greater flexibility and ease of movement. This process has the potential to increase the number of muscle fibres recruited, which can in turn help develop the athlete's strength over time. Reflexively, massage directly or indirectly affects the nervous system. By encouraging relaxation, massage increases the production of endorphins, natural painkillers and mood elevators that create a sense of well-being. In this way, massage may provide psychological benefits that could give the athlete a competitive edge.

The effects of massage can be evaluated both physiologically and psychologically. Evidence supports some of the currently held beliefs, but not enough research has been done to substantiate all of the claims that have been made. As therapists, we obviously believe in the benefits of massage. This belief is a result of historical clinical experience, objective reports and testimonials rather than scientific studies. It is generally believed that the following are some of the effects that massage can have on the body as a whole.

- *Muscular system:* Sports massage can release soft tissue tension, relieve stiffness, decrease muscle spasms, release restrictions and soften and realign scar tissue and loosen up adhesions, helping to restore optimal function.

- *Skeletal system:* By releasing tension and restrictions in soft tissue, it can help to reestablish a balance in muscle function where needed and increase mobility and flexibility, thus reducing the stress on joints.

- *Cardiovascular system:* By increasing blood flow, sports massage brings more oxygen and nutrients to tissue and removes waste products, thus promoting an efficient system.

- *Nervous system:* Massage can stimulate a variety of sensory receptors, depending on the techniques used, to either stimulate or soothe nerves. It can also reduce pain as a result of endorphin release.
- *Lymphatic system:* In general terms massage can help the immune system by promoting fluid movement through the tissue, thus assisting with the elimination of toxins. It is also said to increase white blood cell count to help the body fight disease.
- *Digestive system:* By stimulating the parasympathetic nervous system, sports massage increases digestive movement through peristalsis, thus helping to relieve constipation, colic and gas.
- *Urinary system:* By increasing circulation and stimulating the parasympathetic nervous system, massage improves elimination.

Where Can Sports Massage Take Place?

Sports massage does not require a designated space or need any equipment. You need only your hands and skills to deliver effective massages. At sporting events you can offer pre-event, intra-event and post-event massages. You can offer massages in public places to educate both athletes and non-athletes about the benefits of sports massage in performance and recovery. Sports massage can also be delivered in more formal settings such as multidisciplinary medical centres and health care centres.

Many sports massage therapists set up practices in designated rooms in their homes or provide mobile service. Others offer on-site treatments at offices. Sports massage can be performed almost anywhere—on the floor, at the side of the playing field or in a chair in someone's front room. A broad range of techniques are available, thus allowing you to work with or without lubricant, directly on skin or through clothing. Sports massage is versatile and can fulfill a wide range of needs in a multitude of situations.

When Should Sports Massage Take Place?

Typically, sports massage is used in pre-, intra- and post-event work, as well as being a part of a good training regime (maintenance massage). The duration can be as short as 5 minutes or as lengthy as an hour and a half. (If a massage lasts longer than this, the body can get overloaded, potentially defeating the purpose.) With additional remedial training, you can use sports massage in rehabilitation programs. It can be used in a number of settings such as a hospital or clinic, as part of a physiotherapy treatment or on its own.

When performing sports massage in a pre-event or intra-event situation, be cautious. Unless you have the appropriate skills and adequate knowledge about your client, it is best to leave any deeper or specific work to maintenance massages.

Post-event massage is generally used to return the tissue to its pre-event state; it works with the lymphatic system to flush and aid in normalising tissue. Post-event work can also be an opportunity to assess for any injuries and take the necessary action to ensure a full recovery. Post-event massages are generally gentler and shorter than maintenance sessions. The extent of the massage depends on the type of event; for example, after a marathon, tissues will be tired and lack energy and will not tolerate a vigorous or lengthy massage. Further discussion about event work is given in chapter 10.

Outside of event work, sports massage is for anyone, active or inactive. This form of massage, although it has the word *sport* attached to it, can be suitable for anyone with an interest in soft tissue work who can appreciate the possibilities it has to offer.

CLIENT TALK

When people hear about what you do, many want to talk about their own soft tissue complaints. In situations such as these, you have an opportunity to educate about sports massage and what it can and cannot do. You can also apply some massage through clothing to give the person a feel for your technique. As long as you act responsibly, consider contraindications and do not treat any conditions without doing a full assessment, your hands can act as an advertising and educational tool. Be careful not to give advice until you have taken a full assessment and case history.

Benefits of Sports Massage

The big question is, How does sports massage relate to the real world? How can massage affect an athlete's performance or everyday activity? Whether tension is due to a sporting activity or a job, it can be effectively dealt with through massage. How can you explain this and the possible benefits of massage to prospective clients in a way that will encourage them to include it as an essential part of their lives?

Situation: A swimmer has approached you and asked if you can help him. He has very tight shoulders and is starting to get a bit of lower back discomfort. He also believes his training is not going the way he wants it to despite the time and effort he is putting into it. As a result, he is becoming discouraged about the lack of progress. Your response might go something like this:

'There might be a soft tissue reason for the lack of progress, and a potential one is that you are not necessarily using your muscles efficiently. Sports massage is not just about the feel-good factor; it also addresses how to best maintain optimal performance and prevent injury. We do this by using a multitude of techniques that help muscles perform optimally so they are ready for the demands of sport. By the description you have given, it sounds as though you might have developed some muscle imbalances. We will look at this and determine whether you are creating a high demand for some muscles and not enough for others.

Massage will also increase your awareness through touch. It will show you where your areas of soreness, tension and weakness are. As a result, it will help you to understand how your muscles are behaving and therefore how you might need to adjust your training.

For instance, if the muscles such as the upper trapezius have been overdeveloped and are very short and tight, this will lead to a decrease in the range of motion available to the shoulder. This will have a knock-on effect on the other muscles, inhibiting the other structures and decreasing their ability to assist and support the movement.

This will lead to less available power in the stroke because the full potential of the muscle structures is not being used. Massage will help to keep the fibres lengthened and encourage strong mobile tension in the tissue, developing a more balanced and functional movement.

By keeping the tissues more mobile and not allowing them to stiffen up, massage also encourages the exchange of nutrients and waste products, thereby keeping the tissues healthy. Including sports massage in your training can improve your performance and keep you injury free. I would recommend that you use massage along with your cardiovascular, strength and flexibility training.'

Benefits of Sports Massage

- Greater flexibility and range of motion
- Increased usage of available muscle
- Improved performance
- Improved self-awareness
- Fine-tuning of training
- Functional muscle balance

- Improved fluid movement
- Pain reduction
- Appropriate psychological stimulation (e.g., alertness, clarity, relaxation)
- Greater energy
- Improved recovery
- Injury prevention

Closing Remarks

Sports massage is about treating and meeting the needs of people regardless of whether they are athletes. Anyone who has a soft tissue condition or wants to improve his general well-being or health can benefit from sports massage. As a sports massage therapist, you have a lot to offer, but remember that your work is about meeting the needs of your clients. If that requires that you work alongside other therapies, it is important to be open to these other possibilities. Always consider whether the condition is within your remit of experience and understanding. If not, it is best to seek advice or refer.

Quick Questions

1. Who should be treated with sports massage?
2. How does massage affect the muscular system?
3. When can sports massage take place?
4. What is the main focus of sports massage?
5. What skills do you need as a sports massage therapist?

Contraindications for Sports Massage

In this chapter you will learn the difference between global (sometimes referred to as general) and local contraindications for sports massage as well as the conditions that require application modifications rather than the restriction of massage. To support your understanding of this topic, the Pathology section gives a brief description of common conditions that you might encounter in your practice and some practical approaches about how to modify your massage to accommodate the physiological changes.

Contraindications

Splitting the word *contraindications* offers some insight into its meaning. *Contra* means 'against', as in 'contrary', and *indications* address what can be done. Therefore, contra-indications are conditions that prevent you from continuing. Contraindications are not necessarily absolute. Some situations, referred to as general contraindications, prevent you from applying any form of massage. In the case of local contraindications, you need to avoid specific areas, but you can apply massage elsewhere. Lastly, in some circumstances you will need to make changes or modify your techniques to accommodate the physiological changes in the soft tissue. Adjustments that need to be made as a result of a disease process or condition are classified as modifications.

CLIENT TALK

It is important to have a mentor in your life as a therapist, someone to bounce ideas off of and to help develop your confidence. On numerous occasions my students have come with their clients to seek advice and watch me assess them. I usually give some treatment, but more important, I spend time explaining what I have found and give suggestions as to how they can take over and treat. It can be daunting when you first start working on your own. It is important to feel that you can get reassurances and ask for advice when it is warranted.

Global Contraindications

Global contraindications are conditions that prevent the application of massage globally. The following key words can help you remember all of the conditions in this category: *severe, acute, contagious, uncontrolled* and *undiagnosed*. Although this list is not all encompassing, it will help you determine whether you need to make alternative arrangements such as referring to another health care professional, administering first aid treatment or doing nothing until the situation has changed. Following is a list of some of the most common conditions that are global contraindications:

Alcohol and recreational drugs, such as just having had a glass of wine	Peritonitis
	Phlebitis
Atherosclerosis	Recent surgery
Arteriosclerosis	Severe haemophilia
Acute hypo- or hyperthermia	Severe oedema
Acute injuries (first aid required)	Severe sports injuries
Contagious illnesses such as flus and colds	Severe pain
	Shock
Compartment syndrome	Strong medications
Deep vein thrombosis	Tumours
Heart disease	Uncontrolled hypertension
Inoculations (wait 24 hours)	Undiagnosed lumps

Local Contraindications

Unlike global contraindications, local contraindications allow you to proceed with massage but away from the affected area. Always ensure that what you are doing does not adversely affect the healing process. For example, if your client has a fractured fibula, your considerations should include how to position your client, the choice of techniques and where you should massage so as not to affect the knitting process of the bones. Here is a list of some of the most common conditions that are local contraindications:

Bruises	Hernias	Metal pins and plates
Contusions	Open wounds	Myositis ossificans
Dermatitis	Radiation	Pacemaker
Folliculitis	Severe varicose veins	Tumours
Fractures	Sunburns	Undiagnosed skin disorders
Fungal infections	Melanoma (skin cancer)	Verrucas

Modifications

Modifications require an awareness and understanding of the condition before proceeding. When clients present with underlying conditions, you need to determine how to change your approach to treatment.

To give a safe and effective treatment, you must consider your plan of action prior to the start of the session. At some point during the session, you might need to consider modifications to some or all the following: the choice of technique; whether to work specifically or generally, or superficially or deeply; the direction and speed of the movement; the duration of the massage; the stage of tissue healing; and the positioning of the client.

Consider a client who presents with plantar fasciitis (fascia that is inflamed underneath the foot) as the primary reason for the visit, but also has diabetes mellitus as an underlying issue. You will first need to understand the nature of diabetes before determining how to approach your treatment for the secondary condition. One of the complications of diabetes is that the client can have peripheral neuropathies that can lead to decreased sensation in the feet. Without this knowledge, you may use massage techniques that are too aggressive, unintentionally inflicting more damage to the tissues rather than aiding in the healing process of the plantar fasciitis. In this circumstance deeper techniques such as friction should be avoided; a broader, more superficial soft tissue release stroke in conjunction with stretching techniques farther up the calf would be a safer option to aid in the release of the tension under the foot.

Whenever you are working with diseases or abnormal soft tissue conditions, knowledge about the condition is essential to make the correct modifications to perform safe and effective massage. Always consider that you may need further consultation with a health care practitioner or a doctor's written permission before proceeding with treatment. Following are more examples of conditions that would require massage modification:

Asthma	Frozen shoulder	Osteoporosis
Cancer	Minor surgery	Rheumatoid arthritis
Diabetes	Osteoarthritis	Whiplash

The next section, Pathology, discusses these conditions in more depth.

 If you are unsure about any condition that a client presents with, treat it as a contraindication until you obtain the knowledge you need to proceed in a safe manner for both yourself and the client.

Pathology

Understanding the physiological effects of disease and soft tissue conditions is essential in planning an appropriate treatment. As a therapist, you will encounter a wide range of health issues, and the key to choosing the safest and most effective method for each one will be your knowledge of the condition. As discussed in the Modifications section, some general rules and considerations will enable you to deal with your client's needs. These include the choice of technique, the depth of application, the direction of movement, the duration of the massage, the stage of tissue healing and the positioning of the client.

It is not the intention of this book to give an in-depth explanation of each condition, but rather, a rudimentary explanation of each condition and some guidelines about the role of massage. It is recommended that you include a good pathology book in your library such as *A Massage Therapist's Guide to Pathology, Fourth Edition,* by Ruth Werner or *Clinical Massage Therapy* by Fiona Rattray and Linda Ludwig for further reference.

ASTHMA   Asthma is a reaction to conditions such as stress, pollution or allergens that cause the bronchial smooth muscle tubes to spasmodically constrict. It is associated with local inflammation and excessive mucus production. Signs and symptoms might include wheezing, coughing and difficulty breathing, especially on exhalation. Massage is indicated between attacks to help reduce the stress on the muscular structures that influence breathing. You should pay particular attention to hypertonic intercostals, scalenes, serratus posterior inferior and the diaphragm.

ATHLETE'S FOOT   Also referred to as tinea pedis, athlete's foot is a fungal infection that releases enzymes that digest the keratin in the tissue causing it to split and have a whitish, flaky appearance. This condition loves moist and dark conditions. Fungal infections are highly contagious, yet if you take the correct precautions, you will be able to massage away from the site of the infection. Ask your client to wear a sock during the massage to minimise any risk. Make sure you change and bag the sheets used and disinfect the table using something like diluted tea tree oil.

BUNIONS   Bunions appear on the metatarsal-phalangeal joint of the big toe. They can be caused by a misalignment as a result of an overarched foot, shoes that are too small and pointed, or precipitating factors such as rheumatoid arthritis or a compromised gait. A bunion can look like a large lump with evidence of inflammation. In addition, the big toe can look quite displaced, pushing into the second phalange. Massaging directly on the bunion is contraindicated when it is inflamed. Massage will not decrease the size of the bunion. It is more appropriate to massage the muscles that have had to compensate to avoid the pain in the joint, or to address muscle imbalances that might be going on. A client with a bunion might also need a more supportive shoe, or to be referred to a biomechanical specialist or podiatrist.

BURSITIS   Bursae are fluid-filled sacs that cushion areas where tendons cross over bony angles or provide padding between bony structures. The suffix *itis* indicates an inflammation of the bursa that is painful with both passive and active movements. Massaging directly on the inflamed area is contraindicated, and this is not the best time to try to release the muscles around the area. Although bursitis is not a pathogen that can spread, treatment will have to wait until the inflammation has gone down. In the subacute stage a skilled therapist can work in the area in an attempt to decompress the bones that are affecting the bursa, and soften the muscles that cross over.

CANCER   A very common disease, cancer occurs when normal body cells mutate and replicate malignant cells uncontrollably. Each variety of cancer has specific massage considerations depending on the type and location of the disease. Cancer is no longer considered a contraindication for massage; many now believe that massage can have a positive role in the recovery or treatment of the disease. Treatment depends on the type and stage of the cancer, the goals of the therapy, the types of therapy being used (e.g., radiotherapy, chemotherapy, hormone therapy, surgery) and the age and current health of the client. It is important that you work with the client's medical team in choosing the most appropriate methods of massage treatment.

CARPAL TUNNEL SYNDROME   Carpal tunnel syndrome (CTS) is the entrapment of the median nerve, which is compressed as it passes through the carpal tunnel in the wrist. It can cause numbness and tingling in the hand and usually occurs in those who do repetitive movements for several hours each day. Some types of CTS respond very well to massage, but if the client's symptoms get worse, stop immediately. Favoured techniques are trigger point therapy, fascial techniques and stretching. You can also focus on postural positions and the hypertonic muscles all the way up the arm and in and around the shoulder.

CRAMPS   Cramps are muscle spasms accompanied by intense pain and often occur post-exercise. They can be caused by a decrease in oxygen (ischemia) to the skeletal muscle, low levels of calcium and magnesium, as well as muscle splinting after an injury. Massaging into the belly of the contraction is contraindicated, but working away from it by applying a stretch to the length of the muscle, or engaging the antagonistic muscle to release the protective mechanism, can be effective.

CYSTS   Generally, a cyst is a reaction to something that should not be in the body, much like a pearl, which forms to isolate a grain of sand. In the case of a cyst, tissue surrounds a foreign article or infection to form a mass. Cysts are palpable, usually small, painless masses that move underneath the skin. They are a local contraindication.

DERMATITIS   *Dermatitis* is a general term used for a host of inflammatory skin conditions. It presents in a variety of ways depending on the type of skin reactions that are elicited. Dermatitis is a non-contagious allergic reaction or irritation of the skin. A typical example is a reaction to a substance or plant life. Massage guidelines depend on what the skin condition presents. It is a local contraindication if it consists of boils, is inflamed, has lesions or if the rash can spread. If it is not itchy or the skin is not broken, then massage is appropriate over this area as it will not effect a change in the dermatitis.

DIABETES MELLITUS   Type 1 diabetes is a condition associated with metabolism problems arising from the body's inability to make insulin. Type 2 develops later in life and results in the body being unable to use insulin. This disorder is characterised by the digestive system's inability to metabolise carbohydrates, protein and fat. In both conditions, some of the long-term complications include decreased blood circulation especially to peripheral tissue, which leads to poor healing time and decreased sensation in the injured area as a result of nerve damage. Because of decreased sensation and circulation to the peripherals, you will need to modify the depth and selection of your massage techniques. The skin might be more fragile and have a slower healing capacity. The normal range on the pain scale will not be a reliable measure because the person will have a lessened perception of pain and will feel pressure less strongly. Massage techniques will need to be less invasive or at least modified. If the client has type I diabetes, there will be issues around taking insulin, such as where the insulin is injected, when it is injected, which type is injected and whether it is slow- or long-acting insulin. Massage can affect the uptake of the insulin and the client needs to be aware of this. There is also the likelihood of microtrauma to the tissue at the injection sites. This will require flushing of the area as long as the client has not injected into the area less than one hour prior to massage. When working with people with diabetes, you need to be aware of and recognise adverse reactions such as hypoglycaemia and take necessary precautions.

DISC PROBLEMS   Disc problems can be classified as prolapsed, herniated and slipped discs, whereby the nucleus pulposus or the surrounding annulus fibrosis of an inter-vertebral disc protrudes and puts pressure on the nerve root, the cauda equina or the spinal cord. Symptoms include pain, numbness, muscle weakness and paresthesia. If the client experiences any of these red flag symptoms, then massage is contraindi-cated; refer them to the appropriate health care professionals. Please see the full list of red flag symptoms in chapter 9 under "Pain Assessment" on page 124. Management depends on the presenting symptoms. Most conditions resolve with active rest and pain management. Massage works with the compensation patterns of the soft tissue, creating space for the retreat of any bulging tissue and aiding in relaxing your client due to the effects of pain.

DISLOCATION   Dislocation is a complete separation of the articulating bones in a joint. (Subluxation is a partial separation.) Goals for the treatment of dislocations depend on the stage of the healing process; acute and early subacute stages focus on the medical treatment. Later on in the subacute stage massage can help to untangle the soft tissue scarring enabling a freer range of motion without destabilising the joint. Because a joint can occasionally subluxate or even completely dislocate postinjury, you must take care to position a client so as not to cause undue stress on the area (i.e., if the dislocation took place in the shoulder, then a small towel to support the area when in prone posi-tion would be appropriate; do not move or lift the limb into any stressful positions).

FRACTURES   A fracture is a break in the bone. Local application of massage is contra-indicated immediately and for about 8 weeks after a break, but work done elsewhere is beneficial as long as it does not interfere with the unification of the bone. Initially, you will need to address the musculoskeletal areas stressed as a result of compensa-tion patterns from changes in movement and body placement. After the bone has been allowed to heal for an appropriate time, the soft tissue will benefit from techniques that break down any scar tissue formation. Flushing and reestablishing proprioception and muscle tone to the area should also be a focus. Vibration techniques can be helpful in increasing bone density.

FROZEN SHOULDER   Also known as adhesive capsulitis, frozen shoulder is a restric-tive condition that can be painful and frequently affects the abduction and external rotation of the shoulder joint. Treatment other than massage could entail physiotherapy, medication, surgery, acupuncture, osteopathy, joint mobilisation and exercise. Remedial massage objectives can be divided into three stages. The acute stage is about reducing pain and maintaining range of motion; at this stage aggressive stretches are contraindicated. Massage usually focuses on using reflexive techniques such as NMT, trigger point therapy or positional release. The subacute stage focuses on reducing adhesions (not through friction) and increasing range of motion. This can be accomplished by applying general massage techniques, such as petrissage, as well as STR, MET and gentle stretching. The chronic stage is about restoring full range of motion, addressing scapular stability, stretching to the end of range, doing aggressive glenohumeral joint mobilisation and the reeducation of movement.

HAEMOPHILIA   Haemophilia is a genetic disorder that impairs the blood's ability to clot. The severity of the condition will determine which massage techniques to use and how vigorously to proceed. For the most part, deep, vigorous work (such as frictions) is contraindicated. It is advisable to get medical consent before proceeding with any treatment and to start with a conservative approach (i.e., a short session using gentle techniques, starting off in a more robust area, such as the shoulders).

HEADACHES   Headaches come in a variety of classifications: tension, vascular, chemical and traction-inflammatory. Headaches rarely indicate a serious underlying condition, but if none of the typical triggers are evident, refer clients to the appropriate professionals for investigation. Studies are showing similarities among the various types; however, massage is not indicated for all of them. Generally, only tension headaches respond well to massage, along with a variety of soft tissue techniques. The symptoms consist of steady bilateral pain and can be triggered by muscular tension, ligamentous injury, bony misalignments or musculoskeletal imbalances. Typically, someone suffering with a throbbing vascular headache will avoid massage. Headaches due to central nervous system injuries or infections are contraindications for massage.

HEAT EXHAUSTION   Heat exhaustion can happen when the body accumulates more heat, generated by the muscles, than it can release. This often happens in a marathon when the weather is hot. Symptoms include excessive sweating, dehydration, vasodilation and a headache. Remove the sufferer to a cooler environment. Remove any excess clothing and sponge the person down, being careful not to overcool. Give some sips of water and a salt solution mix (1 tablespoon of salt to 1 litre of water). It's advisable to summon a medical team. Massage is contraindicated.

HEAT STROKE   Heat stroke often follows a prolonged state of dehydration and is the final stage of hyperthermia. It can be fatal if the person's temperature is not reduced to a safe level through immediate treatment. Due to the prolonged sweating, the electrolyte balance will have become critical. This is a serious condition and requires urgent medical attention. Massage is contraindicated.

HAEMATOMA   A haematoma is a pool of blood resulting from internal bleeding; it can appear like a bruise or develop into a sac-like structure. Haematomas that develop into sacs and are not reabsorbed into the body can be surgically removed. Haematomas are a local contraindication for massage.

HYPERTHERMIA   If you are working at events in the summer, you can expect to see various forms of hyperthermia, which is a rise in the core temperature of the body as a result of the hypothalamus not effectively controlling heat levels. There are three stages of heat-related conditions: heat cramps, heat exhaustion and heat stroke, the latter being the most serious. Refer anyone with hyperthermia to a medical aid unit, place the person in a cool environment and encourage the person to sip water. Massage is contraindicated.

HYPOGLYCEMIA   Hypoglycemia is often related to diabetes, but it can be a condition on its own. Simply not eating the right food or not enough of it can cause a low level of blood glucose. Symptoms include dizziness, confusion, chills, sweating, hunger, headache and pallor. The primary concern is to replace fuel. Once symptoms have subsided, massage can be applied.

HYPOTHERMIA   Hypothermia occurs when the rate of heat production is exceeded by heat loss and the body is unable to maintain adequate core temperature. Early signs and symptoms can range from shivering, euphoria, the appearance of intoxication, blue lips and blue nail beds. More advanced signs and symptoms include lethargy, a cessation of shivering, muscle weakness, disorientation, hallucination, combative behavior and unconsciousness. Refer anyone with advanced symptoms to a medical team. Massage is contraindicated.

MULTIPLE SCLEROSIS   Multiple sclerosis can be recognised by its symptoms: fatigue and a loss of sensation, motor control and sometimes vision. It is thought to be an auto-immune disease, but how it is triggered is not completely understood. Multiple sclerosis damages the myelin, the protective sheath surrounding the nerve fibres of the central nervous system, affecting the person's ability to receive messages along the full length of the muscle fibre. Massage is not tolerated in an active stage; it is best to treat during the subacute stages. Overstimulating the muscles during massage could result in activating muscles to painfully spasm. Use flushing techniques to areas that have lost any sensation to maintain mobility to the area. Keep the environment cool to avoid exacerbating symptoms.

MYOSITIS OSSIFICANS   Usually, myositis ossificans follows trauma to the tissue. The injured area that has bled coagulates and calcifies, becoming hardened bone. Normally, when calcification occurs, the body recognises that the calcium deposit is not supposed to be there and reabsorbs it into the body. If the area has not yet calcified then massage is appropriate as long as treatment such as friction is applied to the outer edges of the site and it is not overworked. Massage is locally contraindicated once the area has calcified.

OEDEMA   Oedema is often seen as an increase in fluid in the interstitial spaces of the tissue as a result of circulatory or lymphatic blockages, or electrolyte or protein imbalances. You must determine the causes before developing a treatment plan. Most types of massage are contraindicated especially with systemic oedema because of the impact massage has on the circulatory system. Lymphatic drainage techniques are the therapy of choice; there are those who specialize in this type of massage and would be most suitable for conditions such as lymphoedema. Massage is appropriate in sub-acute situations such as a soft tissue injury or when the client has been immobilised for a period of time.

OSGOOD-SCHLATTER'S DISEASE   Osgood-Schlatter's disease most commonly affects teenagers who participate in sports that involve kicking, running, jumping, turning and twisting actions. Stress is placed on the insertion site of the quadriceps tendon on the tibial tuberosity and can result in swelling, inflammation and possibly a large protuberance. It is a painful condition that can be related to adolescent growth spurts and sometimes obesity. Treatment often consists of easing up on heavy sporting activities, applying cryotherapy and allowing time to do its job. Massage is locally contraindicated at the insertion site of the quadriceps, the tibial tuberosity; however, massage can address the muscle imbalances that might exist due to the growth spurt and offer some ease to areas being overstressed.

OSTEOARTHRITIS   Osteoarthritis is a chronic condition usually found in weight-bearing joints that affects the articular cartilage and subchondral bone whereby the joint structures are irritated and inflamed. This type of arthritis does not usually present itself as acute, but rather, is a chronic condition that responds well to massage. Your goals are to reduce pain by increasing the space in the joint, increasing range of motion through gentle stretching and massaging soft tissue structures that have added to the condition.

OSTEOPOROSIS   A decrease in bone density with a subsequent reduction of structural strength is the definition of osteoporosis. This is usually due to a lack of calcium absorption via vitamin D, as well as endocrine imbalances. Severe osteoporosis is a contraindication, but if there is no evidence of fractures, massage can benefit in a number of ways. As well as helping to alleviate some of the pain, specific techniques such as mild vibration and a cupping style of tapotement can help increase bone density. Avoid any strong pressure directly into the bone or any vigorous work.

PATELLOFEMORAL SYNDROME AND PATELLAR TENDINITIS   Patellofemoral syndrome is a tracking disorder in the knee that causes degenerative changes to the articular cartilage on the underside of the patella. (This can be a precursor to osteoarthritis.) Massage can address the stiffness in the muscle–tendon component of the joint. It is a local contraindication if the area is inflamed. Patellar tendinitis can be confused with patellofemoral syndrome because it affects the same area and has similar painful symptoms. One way to determine whether the person has patellar tendinitis is to ask whether he feels pain when climbing stairs; a person with patellofemoral syndrome hurts when going down stairs. Patellar tendinitis results from the extension of the leg and affects the outside of the joint, whereas patellofemoral syndrome results from the weight of the femur pushing on the patella and affects the inside of the joint. Massage is more effective for patellar tendinitis; the condition responds very well to soft tissue work. Both syndromes benefit from creating a better balance of the muscles.

PLANTAR FASCIITIS   When the plantar fascia underneath the foot becomes inflamed and painful, plantar fasciitis results. The condition is caused from overuse and micro-trauma placed on the fascia, from the degeneration of the plantar aponeurosis, or from both. It is experienced as a sharp, bruise-like pain when placing tension through the foot especially after a period of rest. It eases when muscles are warmed up. Massage can be very effective in releasing the soft tissue tension in the affected structures either directly or indirectly, within pain tolerance. For example, releasing the tension in the superior muscles such as the gastrocnemius can give relief.

POSTOPERATIVE   The safe period to work on soft tissue postoperatively depends on the type and degree of trauma to the area, how well it is healing, client response and the client's current age and health. Any signs of infection or poor healing will prolong any possible massage treatment. Clots are another consideration, because they are one of the biggest causes of death postsurgery. During a subacute stage when there are no signs of inflammation or infection, carefully applied friction around the scar tissue can improve the healing process and realign tissue. Other massage considerations include reflexive work, pain relief, flushing, relaxation and balancing possible compensatory changes in muscles.

RHEUMATOID ARTHRITIS   Rheumatoid arthritis affects women more than men at a ratio of three to one. It is an auto-immune disease that targets the smaller joints of the body, causing inflammation, swelling and the eventual destruction of the joints. Massage is beneficial to maintain as much range of motion as possible, to help flush toxins and to diminish discomfort. If the client is in an acute stage, massage is contraindicated. Start conservatively if it is your first time seeing the client, or it is their first time having massage. Start in a non-affected area using lighter techniques to flush and have a shorter session. Determine the client's tolerance before extending the session or trying more aggressive techniques.

SCAR TISSUE   Scar tissue results when tissue knits or reforms in a disorganised manner after an injury. Collagenous scar tissue is dense, has few blood vessels and lacks pigmentation, hair follicles, normal skin glands and possibly sensory neurons. Considerations for postoperative situations such as healing and signs of infection apply to scar tissue, as do general massage goals. Techniques that are particularly beneficial are friction and soft tissue release followed by flushing with effleurage.

SHIN SPLINTS   Shin splints represent a collection of conditions that include chronic and acute exertional compartment syndromes, tibialis anterior/posterior injury, stress fractures and periostitis. Acute and chronic exertional compartment syndromes are contraindications. Be cautious when working with people with periositis and stress fractures. It is important to determine which type of shin splint they have before proceeding with massage. However, massage on tibialis anterior and posterior conditions works well by stretching and flushing the affected muscles.

SPRAINS   Sprains affect the ligamentous structures that connect bone to bone. The cause of a sprain is usually a sudden wrenching or twisting of the joint beyond its normal range of motion thereby disrupting the stability of the joint. Passive stretching to the affected area will be painful. Healing of a ligament takes longer because of the poor blood supply to the tissue regardless of whether it is a mild, moderate or severe grade of sprain. Proprioceptive work should be included in the massage treatment. Massage and passive stretching in the later stages of the subacute phase is appropriate.

STRAINS   Strains are injuries that affect muscles or tendons. Passive stretching or resisted contraction can cause pain to the affected tissue. Strains can be classified as grade 1 (mild), 2 (moderate) or 3 (severe). Treatment is determined by the stage of the injury and the severity. Treatment for a strain in the acute stage focuses on reducing the signs and symptoms of swelling and pain. In the subacute stage the intention is to normalise the tissue and address the cause of the strain (e.g., poor posture, chronic overuse, previous injuries). The greater the grade of strain, the longer the recovery period will be and the greater the need to seek medical advice. During the acute stage, massage can be applied to areas above the injury site to help flush the area. Massage is more appropriate in and around the injury during the subacute stage. During the early stages of subacute, the focus is more on the flushing techniques. As the tissue heals, deeper techniques to realign the tissue with flushing are appropriate.

TENDINITIS   Tendinitis is a slow-onset, inflammatory condition of the tendon that presents with pain and stiffness and possibly heat and swelling in the acute stage. Pain with resistive movements confirm an injured muscle–tendon unit. In the acute stage, the area should not be directly massaged. The tissue away from the site, however, can be lengthened to reduce the stress to the affected area. In a subacute stage, massage is effective for resolving scar tissue, reducing adhesions and reestablishing range of motion. If your client has recently had a steroid injection for this condition, avoid massage to the area. It will disperse the medication.

VARICOSE VEINS   Varicose veins are abnormally bulging veins that have distended as a result of a weakness in the return valve system. Varicose veins are usually found in the legs. When they occur in other parts of the body, they are known as haemorrhoids, varicoles and esophageal varices. Massage is contraindicated if the person has extreme varicose veins either locally or distally, but those with mild conditions can tolerate a more superficial general massage. Avoid deeper techniques.

WHIPLASH   The term *whiplash* covers a multitude of injuries that can occur with cervical acceleration and deceleration in high-speed sports or traffic accidents. Types of injury include sprained ligaments, strained muscles, damaged cartilage and joint capsules and TMJ problems. In the acute stage, circulatory massage is contraindicated; however, reflexive techniques to rebalance the autonomic nervous system are beneficial for the emotional trauma and shock. In the subacute or maturation stage, massage works well alongside osteopathic or chiropractic treatment.

Closing Remarks

If you are not familiar with, or lack confidence with a presenting condition, err on the side of caution and either refer the person to a more experienced practitioner, to an appropriate medical practitioner or seek advice. At the same time, it is important to take on challenges, do your research and safely experiment with your techniques.

Quick Questions

1. What is the difference between a global and local contraindication?
2. What five keys words are usually associated with a general contraindication?
3. What modifications might you need to make to a massage when presented with any abnormal soft tissue condition?
4. Indicate whether each of the following is a global contraindication, a local contraindication or a modification: flu and colds, acute scar tissue, whiplash, diabetes, cancer, old dislocation of the shoulder, severe pain, open wounds, folliculitis, osteoporosis.
5. What is the difference between a sprain and a strain?

Preparing for Sports Massage

At the start of your career, you may work in a variety of settings. Wherever you end up, you will need to consider common work ethics and set-up protocols, meet the required standards of hygiene and safety and maintain an atmosphere of professionalism.

Venue

Sports massage can take place pitch side during an event, in an open space under a tent with other therapists, in clients' homes or in your own home, offices or in a health care clinic. It is not limited to a space and can be taken anywhere. It is very adaptable and only needs the therapist and their skills.

If you are working in a conventional setting such as a therapy room, your clients' comfort should be your main focus. Consider the environment, what they will see, hear, smell and touch and how it will affect their experience. First impressions are very important, so presenting yourself as a professional from the start is to your advantage.

To get a sense of your venue, travel to your clinic and receive a treatment from a colleague. Take a common route your clients would choose so you can see it through their eyes. Is it accessible by public transport or car? Is parking available? What about the neighbourhood—does it feel safe, clean and inviting? What are your first impressions of the room? Is it warm and clean and does it have an air of professional calmness? Clients will make judgments on the visual aspects of the room, the comfort of the couch, the feel of the towels, background noise and the temperature of the room. All the senses need to be considered. Going through the whole treatment experience will help you see whether anything can be improved.

Before renting a room at a clinic, go in anonymously and ask about the therapies offered. Consider booking yourself for a treatment and ask yourself the questions in the previous paragraph, as well as the following: How does the receptionist greet you? Would you fit in at this clinic? Is the environment conducive to the type of treatment you want to offer? Your impressions can help you determine whether your future clients would want to come to this location.

Table 3.1   Advantages and Disadvantages of Various Settings

Setting	Advantages	Disadvantages
Mobile	<ul><li>No rental cost</li><li>Can take your business to the public (e.g., sporting events, corporate offices, public venues)</li><li>Opportunities to travel with sport teams</li><li>Flexible working hours</li></ul>	<ul><li>More time required to set up and take down, plus travel between clients</li><li>Physically more demanding</li><li>Safety issues</li><li>Location and treatment space not always ideal</li><li>Getting roped into having tea afterwards</li></ul>
External clinic	<ul><li>Wide choice of health or sports clubs, medical and bodywork clinics</li><li>Working alongside other professionals</li><li>Receiving clinical support from other team members</li><li>Receptionist manages appointments</li><li>Usually a couch is supplied along with towels</li></ul>	<ul><li>Competition within the practice</li><li>Some clinics expect you to do your own marketing</li><li>Overhead costs can be high; the clinic can take as much as 50% of the fee</li></ul>
Home clinic	<ul><li>No travel time</li><li>Able to control your environment</li><li>No room rental charges</li><li>Able to claim in your accounts a small percentage of costs (e.g., electricity, heating)</li></ul>	<ul><li>Need to keep the environment clean in all rooms that clients will be able to access</li><li>Decreased personal privacy</li><li>Isolated from other professional colleagues</li></ul>

There are some obvious advantages to working mobile, at your own home or in a clinical setting. The advantages and disadvantages of each are listed in table 3.1. (If you are thinking of working at events, further information about setting up is given in chapter 10.) Consider what your priorities are and what would suit you and your clients best. Most therapists choose a couple of locations to offer their clients choices and to promote themselves to a wider client base.

Equipment

Supplies include a couch, pillows, specialised cushions, couch rolls, hand wipes, towels of varying sizes, lotions, heat and ice packs, an on-site chair and water. These are ideal, but at times in your career you will not have all these luxuries and the only equipment available will be your hands.

Because there is a broad range of equipment to choose from, it can be tempting to go a bit over the top when starting a practice. It's best to begin with the basics and add on as experience teaches you what you need. During your training take the time to try a variety of couches, cushions and lotions. See what works well for you, get feedback from other therapists and make thoughtful choices. Remember, although it is not the equipment that makes the therapist but the quality of the touch, your client's comfort will increase his enjoyment of the session.

Couch

The most important piece of equipment is your couch. Spend some time researching couch suppliers. Obviously, you will want one that will suit your particular needs. If you are going to be a mobile therapist, you will need a portable couch. If other therapists will be using the couch, you may need one that adjusts to various heights and has other adjustable parts. Do you need a face hole? If you are tempted to buy a couch second-hand, try it out first, because comfort is critical and will affect return business. Make sure it has a good amount of padding, is sturdy, has no bits that can potentially break, does not make any noise when a client is on it, is easy to set up, does not have any bars for legs to bang into and of course, meets your needs. The following sections address types of couches and what you need to consider regarding length, width and height.

COUCH TYPE   Following are some issues to keep in mind when shopping for a couch:

- Portable couches are suitable for mobile practices, or if you need to store your couch in a cupboard. They are constructed to be light and easily collapsible. Even though they are light, they are often awkward to carry, especially over any distance. For this reason, it is important to see if you can carry it, keeping in mind that you may have to carry it upstairs or for longer than 10 minutes.

- A couch that adjusts for height can be useful, especially if you are not the only therapist using it. However, most therapists have commented that once they have established their preferred height, they tend not to change it thereafter.

- Couches with face holes give you the ability to apply techniques effectively and are essential for client comfort. Make sure the face hole on your couch is well padded. A massage can be spoiled if the client must constantly adjust her face because the face hole is too hard or the wrong shape.

- Hydraulic couches are obviously suitable only if you have a permanent room. They are sturdy, easily adjustable and present a professional image. If the couch requires electricity, keep in mind that if the mechanism breaks down, or there is no electricity, you are without a couch. Also, the trailing wires can be a safety issue.

CLIENT TALK

I would recommend when buying a couch that you go and test it out yourself. Pick it up and try to walk around to see if you can carry the weight for about 5 to 10 minutes. The weight might be manageable but the awkwardness of the shape might make it a bit more of a challenge. You can solve some of the problem by buying a trolley to pull it, but that does not help you when you have to go up and down a set of stairs, or take it in and out of a car. Also try to assemble and disassemble it, as the hardest part can be trying to flip a bed upright. Finally, lie on it for at least 10 minutes to see if it is comfortable. Pay attention to the amount of padding there is overall and the shape of the face hole. Remember that comfort is part of the experience.

COUCH WIDTH AND LENGTH   In most cases the width of the couch will depend on the height of the therapist and the frame of the client. The standard width of a couch is 24 inches (61 cm). Although a wider couch may be more comfortable for larger clients, it may not be suitable for you because it could force you to lean farther across the couch than your stature allows, resulting in back problems. The standard length of a couch is around 72 inches (183 cm).

TIP   Place a pillow under the ankles of a client who is taller than your couch is long.

COUCH HEIGHT   The correct couch height depends on your comfort. Consider the following general rules when choosing your couch height:

- Client size
- Body part you are working on
- Client position
- Techniques you are using
- Your stance (most important)

Clients come in many sizes and will influence the height of your couch. You will need to lower your couch for larger clients so you can work at your optimum level. If the client is in a side-lying position, the height at the hips will change the working height of the couch anywhere from 5 to 13 centimetres (2 to 5 in.). It is better to have the couch a bit lower than normal height because it is much easier to adjust your height by bending your legs than by lifting yourself up. Chapter 4, Body Mechanics, provides further details on how to determine your ideal working height.

Lubricants

Lotion lubricates your hands as they move across the client's tissue. Too much lotion or the wrong type will interfere with this process. Ideally, try to get a lotion that is not too greasy but soaks into the tissue so you do not have to reapply frequently.

A wide range of lotions are available. Before choosing one, consider the purpose of your massage. If you need to pick up the tissue to affect a change, try a lotion that is not too slippery. If you are doing pre-event work, consider whether the lotion will interfere with anything the client does in the sport, such as holding a racket or contacting opponents. Also, does your client have a preference about whether the lotion has a smell or not? Some people do not like the smell of a perfumed lotion especially when returning to the office. Allergies can be an important factor too. Check your insurance as some carriers will not cover you if you use oil blends and are not trained as an aromatherapist.

CLIENT TALK

Most of my clients have come to accept and like the lotion I use despite its distinct scent. This is partly because they realise that it contains essential oils that aid in the health of the tissue. Some have told me, 'It smells therapeutic'. I also like this particular lotion because it is non-greasy and allows me to pick up the tissue with ease.

If you use too much lotion, your hands cannot get the necessary grip needed to lift and work the tissue. If you do not use enough, you might be in danger of causing too much friction, which could lead to an irritating condition called folliculitis. Ideally, you should be able to push the tissue along without causing the hairs to pull on the skin, but you should also not be able to visibly create a path through the centre of the lotion. Adding more lotion is easier than removing lotion.

If your lotion does not come with a pump, then you must consider the hygiene of putting your hands into a container each time you need more. Remove enough lotion for each session into a separate container. Do not save any of the lotion that is left over from one client to the next.

Direct application of the lotion should be from your hands to the client; do not drip or pour from a container. Pour a bit of lotion into your hands, warm it up and then start to spread it onto your client's skin. Each time you need another infusion of lotion, one of your hands should remain in contact with the client's skin. Either turn the contact hand up to pump more lotion onto it or pump into your free hand. So that you do not break contact with your client, place a number of lotion containers about the room or wear a belt that can hold the container.

Hygiene

It is obviously important to take every precaution not to infect your clients. Infections can be transmitted in the massage environment in the following ways:

- *Direct contact:* A handshake and making contact from one client to another without washing your hands.

- *Indirect contact:* Placing a hand on a doorknob someone else has touched, lying on a towel that has not been washed, resting your face in a face hole that has not been cleaned.

- *Air transmission:* Colds and flu are contraindications for massage. You should not see clients when they are still at a point of ill health and are sneezing and coughing. The same goes for you: If you feel you are coming down with something, cancel your appointments rather than risk transmitting the infection to your clients.

Prevention comes from good hygiene:

- Wash your hands thoroughly with warm water and soap after each treatment.
- Keep your nails short to reduce places for pathogens to harbour.
- Remove all jewellery because lotions tend to accumulate in jewellery, and it can cause skin abrasions.
- Clean in and around the face hole after each client.
- Clean equipment regularly.
- Use fresh towels and a fresh couch roll for each client.
- Keep the room clean and uncluttered.
- Wipe down areas of contact such as door handles.

Client Positioning

Positioning is not just about client comfort. It also helps you access soft tissue structures that would otherwise be difficult. How you move a client from one position to another, how you support the limbs and stabilise the body, how you communicate your instructions—all of these can enhance or detract from the experience of the treatment. Positioning is in itself a skill and requires practice.

Comfort

Comfort relaxes the client, softens the tissue and allows you to work effectively and deeply. An uncomfortable face hole will inadvertently cause tension in the rest of the body. (A simple solution could be to use a face cushion.) Comfort can also come in the form of music, the room's décor, the aroma, the sound of your voice, the feel of the towels and the temperature of the room. A useful way to find out if your treatment space is meeting the needs of your client is to experience it first-hand by receiving a massage using your own equipment. When I did this myself, I was surprised to discover that when a colleague applied the lotion, the room felt so much cooler.

Joint and Limb Support

Joints have limited range of motion. To keep them within their natural range, place pillows appropriately to give support. For example, placing a pillow under the ankles when the client is prone will support the joint and prevent the ankle from being forced into hyper-plantar flexion when you apply downward pressure to the leg. Look out for areas of positional stress such as protracted shoulders while prone. Placing small towels under the shoulders to give support will ease any tension and allow you to work without further stretching muscles that already have too much length to them.

Stability

Always be aware of clients' alignment so as not to compromise their safety. Consider how you can position your client's limbs to maximise stability and how best to place cushions or props to support limbs and joints. A common mistake made in the side-lying position is to incorrectly place pillows and limbs creating an unstable position. Positioning the client's top leg at 90 degrees and making the lower leg straight will create a solid base that will stabilise the pelvis and lower back. (See the photos on page 25.) If you need further stability in the upper body, you can ask the client to hold the edge of the couch in a similar fashion. Place a cushion under the head as well as under the full length of the leg. You can work more effectively with a relaxed, stable client.

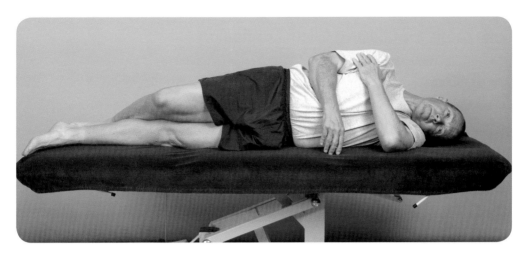

Poor side-lying position.

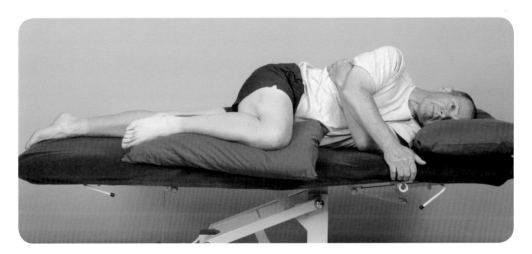

Effective side-lying position with pillows.

Accessibility

At times an alternative position offers better access to a muscle. For example, trying to access the soleus through the thickness of the gastrocnemius can be difficult or uncomfortable for the client. By repositioning a client in a side-lying position, the superficial muscle (gastrocnemius) drops away from the bone increasing the accessibility and making work to the underlying tissue (soleus) much easier.

Four Points for Effective Client Positioning

- Joint and limb support
- Stability
- Comfort
- Accessibility

Positions

You need to give careful thought to maintaining stability and supporting the limbs when moving a client into a new position. Towel control is equally important during this process. The various positions include supine, prone, side-lying and sometimes sitting.

SUPINE POSITION Place a pillow under the head and knees for support. (A bolster can also be used under the knees.) This allows the body to rest in a natural position while giving ease to the lower back. Placing a pillow behind the knees also prevents the joint from being forced beyond a normal range of motion during massage.

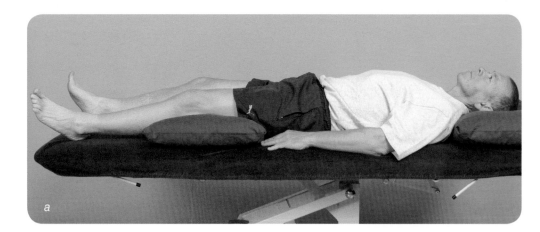

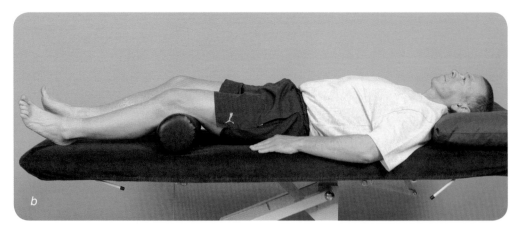

Supine positioning using *(a)* a pillow under the knees and *(b)* a bolster under the knees.

PRONE POSITION   Placing a cushion under the torso or pelvis is optional. If the person is severely lordotic or has lower back issues, offering support to this area is important. Large chested women might also need a cushion under their torso to even things out a bit. Placing a cushion under the ankles prevents excessive flexion of the ankle and foot. Place small towels or cushions under the shoulders for clients with protracted shoulders or for those that are large chested.

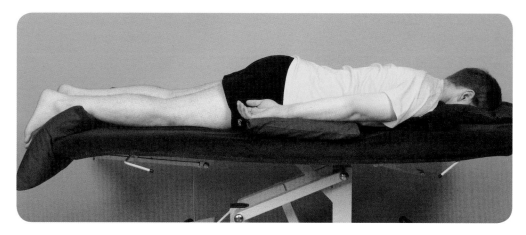

Prone positioning.

SIDE-LYING POSITION   Pay particular attention to the alignment of your client in a side-lying position. It is easy to get this incorrect and place him in an unstable position. Making sure that the client's top leg is at 90 degrees and the lower leg is straight will help to stabilise the pelvis and lower back and keep them in alignment to one another. If the client needs further stability in the upper body, ask him to hold the edge of the couch. Place a cushion under his head as well as along the full length of his leg. See the photo earlier in this chapter on page 25 for proper side-lying positioning.

SITTING Sitting is a useful position but potentially an unstable one. Make sure the client's feet are able to rest flat on the floor as he sits on the edge of the couch. To offer support for the back, place a pillow between you and the client.

Having a chair on site can be useful. A chair is mobile and does not require a lot of room, and the massage can be done through clothing. A chair also supports your clients without placing undue stress on the back. This is particularly useful for clients who have back problems and find it difficult to get onto a couch. You will need further basic training in order to work with clients in this position.

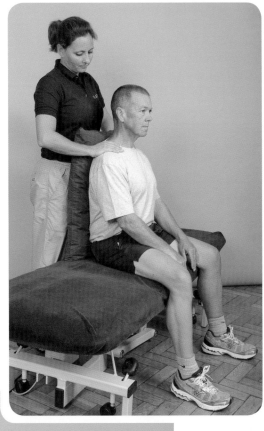

Sitting position on a couch.

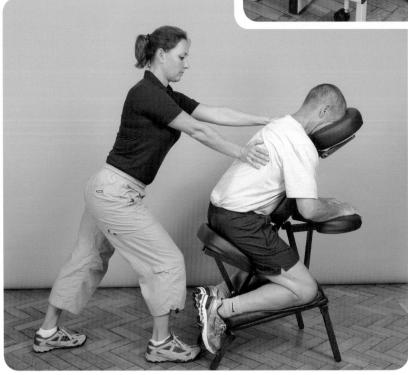

Sitting position in an on-site chair.

Towel Control

Maintaining towel control while moving a client takes practice. Here are some simple rules that will help you accomplish this with confidence:

1. Minimise the number of towels you have to control; it's best to use one large one.
2. Make sure the towel is covering the client in such a way as to maintain modesty.
3. Remove cushions from the couch before moving the client.
4. Hold the towel with your thighs on the side closer to you.
5. Place your hands far apart on the opposite side and lift the towel slightly.
6. Give clear instructions when directing your client to move.

When changing a client's position, you have several options in controlling your towels. To simplify things, two approaches are presented here. The first demonstration is easier when first starting out; it does not require you to anticipate which direction your client will move. The second demonstration (on page 30) requires you to be more intuitive about the direction your client will move, but the towel control is more fluid once you have mastered which end to hold down in order to maintain control. If you misjudge the direction, the towel will go with the client, leaving you both embarrassed.

Place yourself close to the couch. Press your legs against the side of the couch to hold the towel in place. Avoid holding your towel too high or too low; lifting the towel to the correct height allows the client to move freely and maintains modesty. Make sure you hold the towel at both ends, far enough apart to ensure the client's modesty is maintained throughout the process.

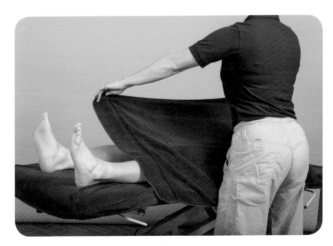

Holding the towel with the thighs.

In the process of a client's repositioning, you will need to ensure one of two things: Give very clear instructions about which direction you would like the client to turn, or become very proficient at anticipating which direction a client will turn. Either way, you will need to hold the towel at either end to ensure the important areas remain covered.

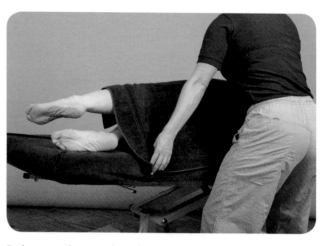

Picking up the towel on the opposite side.

Sometimes, despite giving clear instructions, a client will mistake left for right and right for left. When this happens, stay responsive to the situation. As you progress and become more confident as a therapist, moving your clients and changing their positions during a session will become a regular routine and you will be able to perform it with ease. Developing this skill will give you greater access to more muscles in a number of positions while maintaining clients' modesty. This skill will be vital when performing tests as well as applying more advanced positions (e.g., a leg raise in supine).

TIP When you are first starting out, try moving someone who is fully clothed from one position to another, so mistakes are humorous rather than embarrassing. Also, try a couple of towel techniques and see which one suits you best.

Safety

The safety of your clients is a priority both in terms of the room and equipment and their general well-being. If after a treatment your client is in no condition to get herself to where she is going, alternative arrangements should be made.

CLIENT TALK

Near the end of a massage treatment, it became evident that a diabetic client of mine was not able to get herself home. Although she had taken her morning insulin, she had failed to eat adequately before treatment. By the end of the session she was clearly in distress and needed immediate treatment. Once her sugars had been stabilised and she was in a more cognitive state, I arranged for her daughter to pick her up. Even though she was stabilised, she was still not 100 percent; it was better to err on the side of caution.

Although basic first aid training is not always required for sports massage therapists, it is highly recommended, especially if you are involved in sports with a high risk for on-site injury. You should also always have a first aid kit available and know how to use it. It should include scissors, non-latex gloves, gauze pads and roll, compresses, adhesive tape and adhesive bandages. (Make sure to check periodically to see whether anything has expired.)

It is also wise to practise good environmental safety protocols, such as the following:

- Regularly maintain and check all of your equipment.
- Make sure no articles of clothing are left on the floor that would interfere with movement around the couch.
- If your couch is on casters, ensure that the brakes are engaged.
- Keep the door to the room unlocked.
- Provide regular maintenance and attend to all areas of use including walkways and parking.

Closing Remarks

In the beginning there appears to be a lot to do and many decisions to make before you even start massaging. This is true, and getting this right is essential because it constitutes the foundation of your practice. If you are not properly prepared, your clients will sense this and may not return.

Quick Questions

1. What are the advantages of working in a clinical setting?
2. What are three ways to transmit infection?
3. What are your priorities when positioning a client?
4. Where can pillows be placed when a person is in a prone position?
5. Why is it important to put a pillow under the knees of a client in a supine position?

Sports Massage Techniques

The chapters in part II prepare you to apply techniques in a manner that will prolong your career as a massage therapist. All who work in the field of physical healthcare need to consider their method of practical application so they can both protect their own posture and be safe and effective with their clients. Chapter 4 walks you through appropriate body mechanics as well as correct couch height, working postures and principles of application. The Quick Questions at the end of the chapter help to reinforce your understanding of the material.

Chapter 5 demonstrates the massage techniques that are the foundation of sports massage. Although these techniques are used in many forms of massage, they are unique in the context of sports massage because of how and where we apply them. The pictures and accompanying explanations serve as both visual teaching aids and references and are suggestions, not absolutes. The intention is to give you ideas from which to develop your own techniques. Allow yourself to alter or adjust positions so you are more comfortable while adhering to the principles suggested for effectiveness and safety. The chapter offers numerous helpful hints to ensure that you understand these principles, and the Quick Questions at the end of the chapter reinforce the information.

4

Body Mechanics

Good body mechanics is the foundation of all practical massage techniques. It determines your ability to work with ease and have a long career free of personal injury. A common cause of therapist failure is the misunderstanding and incorrect application of leverage and alignment. Effective application will also result in greater control and power in each stroke, which in turn will attract a returning client base.

Body mechanics is also about applying the 'feel' of the massage in a controlled way. Clients want a massage that has the right depth, neither too light nor too strong. As a therapist you are trying to meet those needs by working in cooperation with the tissue. By following the principles of leverage and proper alignment, you will be able to work in an optimal, safe manner.

Massage Couch Height

Choosing the right couch is the first step in ensuring you are able to work at a comfortable and effective level. As discussed in chapter 3, there are various considerations to keep in mind before buying a massage couch. Once you have the couch, you may need to adjust the height based on the following criteria to achieve proper body mechanics:

- *Size of your client:* The structure and body size of a client will play an important role in the placement of your arms away from your body. To get the angle right for a larger person, you will need to lower the bed.

- *Area of the body you are working on:* Choose the thickest part of the body, usually around the pelvis and abdominal area, to judge the correct angle of your arms.

- *Position of your client:* There is a substantial height difference between the hip in a side-lying position and the thickest body part in a prone position. Hence, you will need to lower the bed to accommodate the side-lying position.

- *Technique you are using:* The ability to adjust the height of the couch becomes more critical when you are working with advanced techniques and need to move your client around in order to perform the technique. At the start of your training you are more likely to adjust your leg position in order to work effectively rather than adjusting the bed or your client.

■ *Your stance:* Your legs are the key to controlling the depth and speed of your work. The ideal position is to stand with your feet approximately 90 centimetres (3 ft) apart, which will lower your stance.

CLIENT TALK

When first starting out, most therapists buy a good mobile bed until they are more established and can install a more permanent one, such as a hydraulic couch, which can be adjusted with ease to make it easier to move the client around. You can usually make enough of a height change by adjusting your legs rather than the couch. For instance, tapotement is best applied if you keep your forearms at a right angle to your upper arms. The easiest way to do this is to bend at the knees to lower yourself down to the right height rather than adjusting the bed.

It is better to have a couch that is too low than one that is too high, because you can adjust yourself by bending your legs or widening your stance to get lower while still maintaining the depth and control of the movement. It is important that you maintain your alignment as well; otherwise, you will put a strain on your back by bending forward. Conversely, if the couch is too high, you will stress your shoulders and upper body.

TIP Adjust couch height based on the size of your client, the body part you are working on, the position of your client, the technique you are using and your stance.

Working Posture

To develop the most effective working posture, apply the following principles:

■ *Keep your shoulders and hips squared into the direction of the stroke.* This permits the energy to come from your legs without any rotational movement, which could put stress on your lower back.

■ *Adopt a wide stance.* This allows you to move more freely.

■ *Place your arms away from your body approximately 30 degrees.* This allows you to generate momentum from your legs and through your body. It also prevents you from squishing muscle into bone.

■ *Create a circle with your arms.* Circling enables you to work efficiently, applying power and strength without effort.

■ *Keep your arms lengthened without locking out your elbows.* Bending your arms too much will interrupt the alignment of your body and inhibit any strength from coming from your legs.

■ *Generate movement from the legs and not the arms as much as possible.* This keeps your arms relaxed, which results in a strong touch that is not invasive or pokey. Unnecessary tension in your upper body, arms or hands is transmitted into the stroke.

■   *Maintain long levers.* As an overall approach to movement and your positioning, try to imagine a long pole that starts at the base of the feet and then moves through the hips to the top of the head. This is an ideal posture for generating force, but it does not mean you cannot bend your joints. The idea is not to collapse into the movement by bending too much, but to keep as long a lever system as possible through your arms, hips, torso and legs (see the two photos that follow). This allows the whole of the body to work together rather than a portion of a limb or body part working independently (e.g., if you bend too much at the waist it will put pressure on the lower back and prevent most of the power from being generated from the legs through the arms). It also changes the quality and depth of the stroke, so when you want to go deeper, you will be forced to use a lot more effort in the upper body in order to increase your depth. If you have the technique right you will find it easy and will not tire.

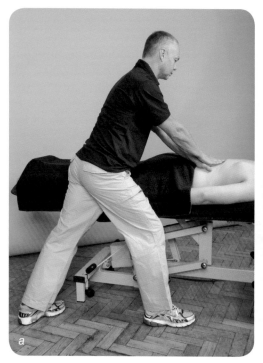 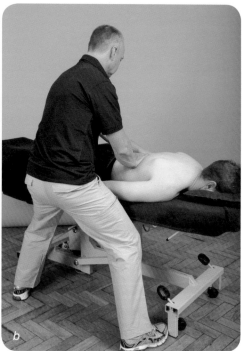

Effective working postures: *(a)* asymmetrical and *(b)* symmetrical alignments.

TIP Following are the principles of a safe and effective working posture:

- Keep your hips and shoulders squared
- Adopt a wide stance
- Place your arms away from your body
- Maintain long levers
- Create a circle with your arms
- Do not lock your elbows
- Generate movement from your legs

Principles of Application

Now that you have established the correct height of your couch and a basic working posture, here are some other methods that are essential to an effective working approach.

CLIENT TALK

To assist you in becoming more sensitive to the tissue underneath your hands, try not to look at what you are doing but allow your hands to transmit the information to you. By changing the focus to your hands, you increase the sensitivity of the touch receptors in your fingers, which in turn will give you more accurate information about the tissue. Using the eyes is a bit like trying to look through a smoked glass window. The other added benefit to not looking at what you are doing is that it helps with your ability to maintain an upright posture: The head is no longer dropping and pulling your shoulders down towards your work.

Asymmetrical Alignment

Working asymmetrically creates a balance between your upper and lower body, and from side to side. In this position it is much more efficient to use techniques that require you to push away from yourself (e.g., long strokes, effleurage). Try to keep your eyes looking forward rather than down. This will help you maintain an upright posture. Over time you will get a good sense of where your hands are and what structures you are feeling and will not need to look. When choosing a different body part to work on, maintain the asymmetrical alignment. (See page 36 for an example of asymmetrical alignment.)

Symmetrical Alignment

A symmetrical stance is when both feet are placed out to either side while the hips are facing forward. The feet should be slightly more than hip-width apart with knees slightly bent. This position is more useful when you are using gathering techniques such as petrissage. To generate movement from your legs, try to rock from side to side or push up from bent legs. To help support your torso, engage your abdominal muscles as you gather and lift the tissue towards you. For an added variation, allow your hip and torso to slightly push your arms forward and pull them back; in other words, while one side of your body is pushing one arm, the other side of the body is pulling the other arm back. (See page 36 for an example of symmetrical alignment.)

Movement

The key to applying a really dynamic stroke is an awareness of how you use your body as a whole. Imagine a long piece of string that goes from your foot to your head; when you pull on one end, it causes the other end to move. Apply this to how you move about while massaging. Consider where the power is being generated from. What part of your body is actually doing most of the movement, and what part of your body tires first?

Try this awareness exercise and observe how you move (i.e., what moves and what does not move). Start by getting into your stance and close your eyes (this allows you to have a greater sense of where the movement is coming from). Choose a stroke and perform it. What generated that movement? Did your arms move first, or did your feet initiate the movement?

Ideally, you should allow the lower portion of your body (i.e., your feet) to generate the movement throughout the length of your stroke. Try your stroke again, but this time do not let the arms move unless the feet are leading the movement and the arms are following. You might need to practise this a few times, but be persistent. By using your body in a connected way, you will be able to control the depth, the power and the flow of your strokes.

TIP Try to let your legs lead the movement in both asymmetrical and symmetrical positions. If you feel that your legs are moving further than your arms or visa versa, then they are working independently of one another. Whatever range of movement the legs have the arms should be moving in tandem and the same distance.

TIP Principles of effective movement include the following:

- Ease versus effort
- Self-awareness
- Eyes forward
- Asymmetric alignment
- Symmetrical alignment
- Increasing the angle
- Unity of movement
- Equal exertion

Increasing Depth

Whenever you intensify a stroke, stay in tune with the reaction of the tissues under your hands and get feedback from your client. A general rule is: The deeper you go, the slower you should move. Indicators that you are moving too fast can be the muscle pushing you out by contracting and becoming tense or your client's verbal response, a fidget elsewhere or a clenched fist. Physiological symptoms might include an overall light perspiration or reddening of the ears. It is important to work in cooperation with the tissue. A certain amount of discomfort may be necessary and welcome; the client will indicate if it is good pain or bad. (See chapter 9 for more information about pain assessment.) To increase the depth of your stroke, you can bring your body over the movement or use a different form of an already familiar stroke.

Increasing the Depth of the Stroke

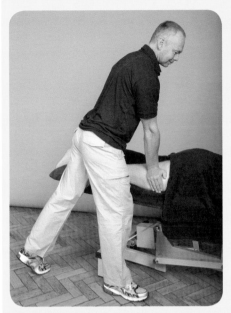

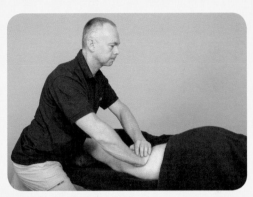

Using assisted hands.

Bringing the body over the movement.

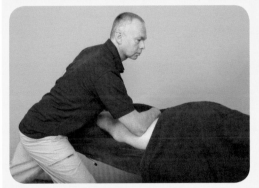

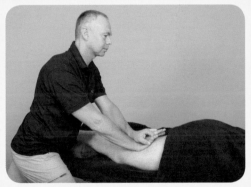

Using the forearms.

Using the heels of the hands.

Other ways to increase the depth of your stroke include generating power from your legs and changing the angle in which you apply the stroke. Consider a situation in which you want to address the deeper tissues of a rather large athlete who has a strong build. Bringing your upper body over the movement to produce more force is very effective. Be careful not to create too severe an angle in your wrist because this stresses the joint and could lead to a repetitive strain injury.

SELF-ASSESSMENT OF THE PRINCIPLES OF APPLICATION

Answer the following questions to evaluate how well you are applying the principles of good body mechanics. The easiest way to do this exercise is to ask someone to observe you and answer these questions.

Is your back in line with your hips and legs?	Yes	No	Are you bending at the waist?	Yes	No
Are you looking straight ahead?	Yes	No	Are you looking at what you are doing?	Yes	No
Are your shoulders relaxed?	Yes	No	Are your shoulders elevated?	Yes	No
Are your arms in front of you?	Yes	No	Are your arms at your side or close to the body?	Yes	No
Is your breathing easy and relaxed?	Yes	No	Are you holding your breath or sweating?	Yes	No
Are you pushing from your legs?	Yes	No	Is the momentum coming from your upper body?	Yes	No
Are your arms relaxed?	Yes	No	Are your arms or hands shaking?	Yes	No
Are you able to physically cope?	Yes	No	Are your joints or muscles showing signs of discomfort?	Yes	No

- If you answered yes to all of the questions in the left column, well done! You are practising good body mechanics.
- If you answered yes to any of the questions in the right column, you need to revisit the principles of application.

From S. Findlay, 2010, *Sports massage* (Champaign, IL: Human Kinetics).

Closing Remarks

As much as possible, keep to the working posture principles presented in this chapter. At times you may need to work with just one arm, open up your hips or rotate your torso. If these situations are infrequent, they will not have any long-term effects. Although the working posture principles in this chapter will minimise your risk of injury, as in sport, repetition over time can cause injury. If you take care of yourself by keeping fit, stretching, having a regular massage (no, not once a year) and being proactive about your health, you should remain injury free.

Quick Questions

1. What are the seven principles of a safe and effective working posture?
2. If you have any discomfort during or after massaging, what should you do?
3. What is the general rule of thumb when applying a deeper stroke?
4. What are some of the symptoms a client will display if the depth of the stroke is too strong or fast?
5. From what principle area is the depth of a stroke generated?

5

Massage Techniques

The fundamental sports massage techniques originated from Swedish massage (effleurage, petrissage, compression, vibration and so on). Over time, additional tools have been added such as muscle energy techniques, myofascial work and neuromuscular techniques, which have come from other bodywork professions such as osteopathy and physiotherapy. This has led to the remedial techniques of sports massage. Learning the massage strokes in this chapter will form the basis of your training. (See the table on pages 63-64 for a summary of the massage techniques discussed in this chapter.) No matter how many other techniques you go on to learn, these basic soft tissue techniques will always be some of the best and most appreciated by your clients.

Components of a Massage Stroke

When first learning how to apply massage strokes, you will need to consider the following technical components of massage. These will help you develop effective application methods before you start.

DIRECTION   The choices of direction are longitudinal, transverse and circular. All strokes in all directions can be used on the torso, but longitudinal strokes applied to the peripherals should be deeper and stronger towards the heart and significantly lighter on their return. This is to mirror and work with the venous lymphatic return system. Transverse is also suitable for legs and arms. If you are using a smaller stroke such as friction, small, circular movements will not interfere with this system.

PRESSURE   Initially, you should apply light, superficial pressure to warm up the tissue and prepare it for deeper work as well as to assess the condition of the tissue and determine which areas need attention. Once the tissue has been sufficiently warmed up, you can apply deeper strokes. During and at the end of a treatment, it is always beneficial to flush the section that you have worked on as well as the surrounding tissue using effleurage.

Regardless of the degree of pressure you are using, you should massage in a thoughtful manner, feeling the various tissues under your hands and reacting to any adverse tension. Areas of tension might require you to slow down and ease off the pressure to get a favourable response. The deeper you go, the slower you should go. Following are areas that require less pressure:

- Bony prominences (e.g., vertebrae)
- Areas of less muscle mass (e.g., shins)
- Areas of greater sensitivity (e.g., chest)
- Areas that have underlying sensitive structures (e.g., the femoral artery behind the knee)

THERAPIST'S TOOLS   The therapist's tools consist of the heel of the hand, fingers and thumbs (reinforced), assisted hand, fists, forearms and elbows. (Look ahead for basic techniques.) Elbows should be introduced after you have more experience and can use them with sensitivity. The most important consideration is to protect your hands and not to overuse them or hold tension in them. It is well documented that therapists with poor technique have short careers as a result of repetitive strain injuries that affect their hands, arms, shoulders and lower back.

Basic Techniques

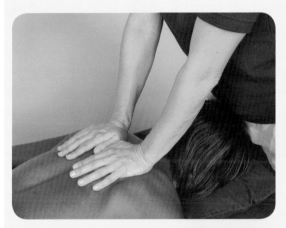

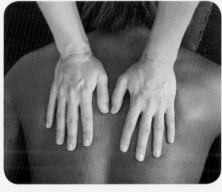

Heel of hand.

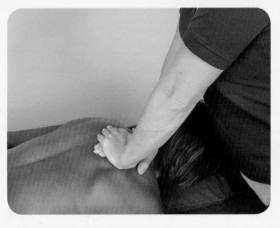

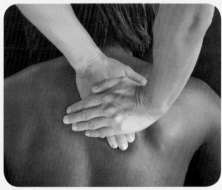

Reinforced fingers.

»continued

Basic Techniques »*continued*

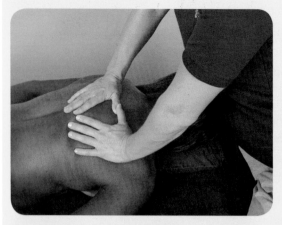

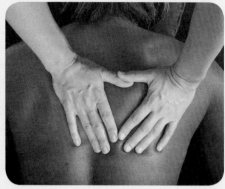

Reinforced thumb.

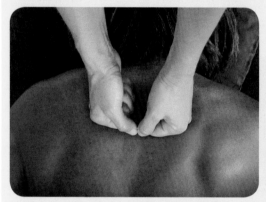

Fists/knuckles.

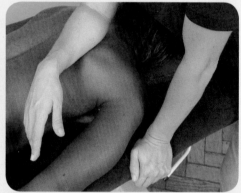

Forearm.

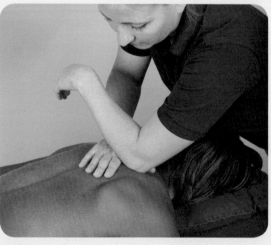

Elbow.

The hands are the most important tool in a therapist's kit. They are sensitive, dexterous and versatile and can transmit all kinds of information about the condition of the tissue. When you start to train, from the first time you place your hands on a client, let your hands take over from your eyes. Hands tell you more than eyes do. If you have difficulty not looking at what you are doing, try either closing your eyes or wearing a blindfold initially to practise and get comfortable with the feel. Further information about movement and seeing through your hands can be found in chapter 4.

Avoid using your thumbs as much as possible. Allow them to be passive partners to your hands. It is possible to use the thumbs for specific work without putting excessive force through them or tensing them up during a movement and still be effective. How you accomplish this will be explained in the relevant technique sections.

RHYTHM AND SPEED   The deeper you go, the slower your strokes should be. The intent is to work with the tissue, meeting the resistance, not forcing your way through. Do not rush or be jerky with your strokes; keep the same rhythm throughout the whole length of the muscle and avoid any flicking actions at the end of the stroke. A smooth transition from one stroke to another encourages the muscles to remain relaxed. Maintain a rhythm that makes it hard for the client to know when you change techniques.

LOCATION   The area of the client's body that you are working on will influence your choice of method, stroke, speed, direction and depth. For example, when working on the chest, there are a few more restrictions with regards to the direction of movement, placement of hands, and depth. Additionally, there is more to consider to maintain client modesty than, for example, working on the legs. Consider the following:

- When working on the chest of a female client, maintain modesty by working above the towel line which should be above the upper half of the breast. Keep your gaze looking away from the chest as this can be very intimidating. Placing your hands and moving in an appropriate direction is also important for maintaining a client's modesty.

- The area available to work on can restrict your choice of tools (e.g., hands versus forearm). If your hands are large and the area you are working is small, you may need to make further adjustments. You may only be able to use the fingers rather than the heel of the hand.

- The soft tissue can be very sensitive. Therefore, you will need to use a slower speed.

- On most people the depth of the muscle is not very thick; therefore, too much force can be an issue.

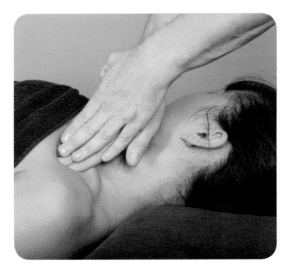

DURATION   A common therapy mistake is over enthusiasm. Therapists sometimes have the idea that they need to fix everything in one session. Unfortunately, tissue does not usually react favourably if it is overworked. Less is more; doing less allows you to gauge the reaction and tolerance levels of the tissue.

Initially, apply your techniques in a general fashion, becoming more specific as the tissues warm up. Apply an appropriate range of techniques to the area until you feel a change in the tissue, which might be a small one, then finish with a general flush to the area. You may only need a few minutes to effect a change.

Other considerations include the current health of the client and the tissue's stage of healing. With clients who have pre-existing diseases (e.g., diabetes) that might slow down or interfere with the healing process, do less and monitor their reactions; then reevaluate and increase the length of time, depth, area worked on, etc. This will help you determine their tolerance to massage and its effects.

TIP Following are some application tips:

- Avoid looking
- Remember that slower is better
- Start superficially, move into deeper work and finish with superficial strokes
- Support your digits
- Avoid using your thumbs
- Keep your hands relaxed

- Work in a general manner, move on to more specific work and finish with general flushing strokes
- Maintain rhythmical movements
- Flow from one technique to another
- Generate movement from your legs

A general misconception is that massage requires considerable physical work and effort. If you apply the principles from chapter 4, massage for the most part should be effortless.

With practice, the individual components and strokes will begin to flow together and connect seamlessly. At the start it can feel foreign and unconnected. Keep revisiting each of these components, reviewing and reassessing your movements. Get honest feedback from those you practise on. For more specific feedback, seek out those who have gone through a form of massage training and can give you technical advice. You can also learn a great deal from receiving a massage. Experience different types of massage from a number of people from whom you can pick up ideas and of whom you can ask questions.

CLIENT TALK

Based on experience, whenever I have felt my stroke has been awkward, or simply does not feel good to me, it will be the same for the client. Massage should always be enjoyable to both of you. If what you are doing feels good to you, it will more than likely feel good to your client.

Effleurage

Effleurage is the technique you begin a massage with and return to throughout. It has a vast range of purposes and effects that make it a very versatile and important technique. Effleurage can be applied both superficially, which tends to have a reflexive value, and deeply, which has a more mechanical one. Effleurage is for spreading the lotion and warming up the tissues. It creates a calming, relaxing effect both physiologically and psychologically, or it can stimulate depending on the speed of application. It is one of the principal forms of superficial and deep evaluation. It is used as a connecting technique from one stroke to another and functions as a flushing procedure to assist general circulation and the return of lymphatic fluids.

TIP The purposes of effleurage:

- Introductory technique
- Warming up
- Spreading the lotion
- Flushing

- Calming or stimulating
- Connecting strokes
- Palpation and assessment

To perform effleurage, keep your hands relaxed. If you are stiffening up, shake your hands out to make them floppy and soft and place them like this onto the body, trying to keep this softness throughout your movement. Your power and strength should come from the lower half of your body. (Refer to chapter 4 for more on proper body mechanics.) Most of the energy should transmit through the heel of your hands, followed by slight tension in your fingers. Your thumbs should remain predominantly passive. The direction of the stroke is classically longitudinal, with the deeper application being towards the heart followed by a significantly lighter returning stroke. This rule applies when working on the peripherals. Alternative directions include transverse and circular. You can return to effleurage throughout the massage. To perform a deeper effleurage stroke, increase the pressure, or power, from your legs (also, see the Deep Strokes section later in the chapter).

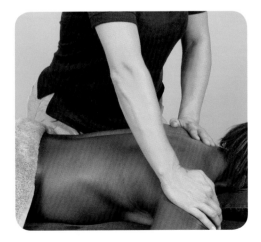

Longitudinal effleurage stroke.

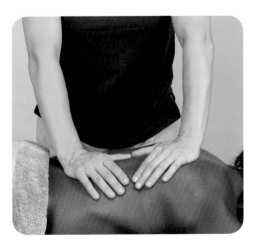

Transverse effleurage stroke.

Petrissage

Petrissage is from the French word *petrir,* which means 'to knead'. It is a deeper stroke than effleurage and often follows it. It includes movements such as kneading, skin rolling, lifting, squeezing and stripping. Like effleurage, the direction and pressure of the stroke varies.

TIP The purposes of petrissage:

- Deeper stroke
- Separating tissue, loosening adhesions
- Relaxation or stimulation

Petrissage is best applied by involving your whole body in the movement and not just your arms or hands. By getting the lift to come from your legs and the gathering action from your abdominal muscles, you will transmit less physical stress through your shoulders and arms. When using the various forms of petrissage, avoid any overuse of the thumb. It should be saved for times when you need to do more specific work, such as for friction or deep strokes. For the most part, your thumbs should remain passive and follow through the movement, playing a supporting role rather than a leading one.

Create a circular position with your arms, keeping your elbows out and arms well in front of you, maintaining an upright position. Using a symmetrical position and moving the legs slightly from side to side, gather the tissue towards your opposite hand. To do this same stroke on the legs, your hips will need to pull back and push forward to generate the movement of your arms creating more of a transverse stroke rather than a longitudinal one. Although you have changed direction, this still allows you to work with the circulatory system of the legs since you are not working against the flow.

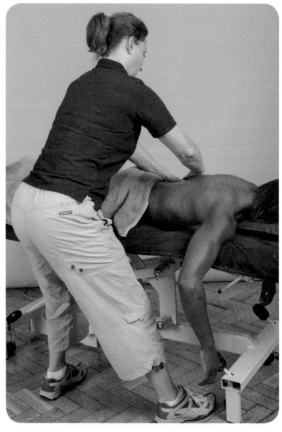

Circular petrissage stroke on the torso.

The pressure from one hand going towards the midline needs to match that of the other hand coming in the opposite direction; otherwise, you will pull the client's leg off the couch. Alternatively, you can hold the client's leg with one hand while applying the stroke with the other. It is more useful to stand feet wide apart in a symmetrical stance when applying this technique. In this position you can generate your power from your torso and hips through to your hands by making the pushing and pulling action come from them. Avoid using the shoulders as this will cause you to twist through the upper back putting undue stress there.

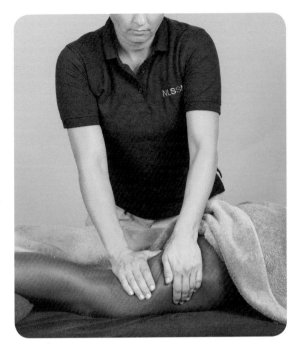

Wringing.

Kneading can be likened to working with dough. It consists of manipulating the tissue in a number of ways—lifting, squeezing, moving it in a circular fashion or working transversely. This technique is versatile and has the fewest application rules.

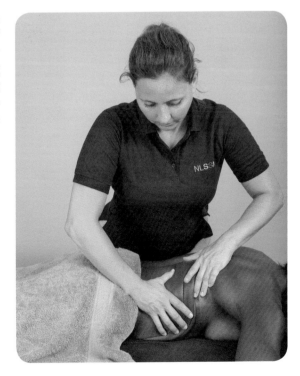

Kneading.

Compression

Compression can be used throughout a regular massage as well as at sporting events as a dry technique to warm up muscles and increase blood flow. It can also be applied through clothing or a towel and is convenient to use at an event when an athlete has a lot of gear on and cannot remove it. It can be used following the application of a deeper stroke to relax a muscle that has tensed up. Compression is a bit like the action of a sponge; squeezing pushes out the fluid, and releasing sucks up more fluid. This pumping action helps to flush the tissues.

TIP The purposes of compression:

- Dry technique
- Warming up
- Flushing
- Relaxing

- Deactivating hypertonic muscles
- Targeting other receptors
- Deactivating muscle spasms

Apply compression at an angle of around 45 degrees; this ensures that you are not pressing the soft tissue into the bone, but are administering a comfortable pressure and then releasing it. The depth depends on the intention (superficial versus deep) and the area you are working on. For instance, because the gluteus muscles are deep and strong, they can tolerate a lot of force; the arms cannot tolerate as much. To work more superficially, lessen the pressure transmitted from your foot and decrease the angle of your stroke. The gluteus muscles are the largest and deepest for this technique and can take a fair amount of pressure, but always check with your client to gauge their comfort level. One method for deep compression is to apply your technique using your fist. Ensure your wrist is in alignment with the arm; you can use the other hand to reinforce the wrist and to help control the movement. Remember, the power is coming from your legs through the alignment of your torso and arms.

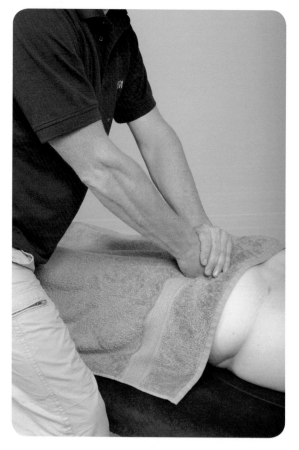

Compression on the gluteus muscle.

Alternatively, you can use a variety of positions to drop the muscle away from the bone, squeezing and lifting away. For example, sit on the bed in an upright position. Taking your elbows out, use the heel of your hands to apply pressure to the calf muscles away from the bones. Press and release working your way down towards the knee, remembering that the direction of blood flow is towards the heart. This position is only suitable if the dimensions of your body and your client's is similar. If you find you are slouching in order to rest their foot on your shoulder choose an alternative method of application. Be aware that by doing this type of squeezing and lifting that you are pressing one hand towards the other and that the tissue can still get squished as the hands take on the role of the bone and become the counteracting force in the movement.

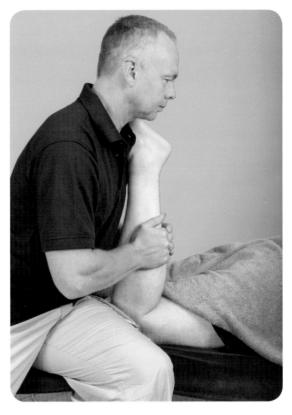

Dropping the gastrocnemius away from the bone.

Deep Strokes

Deep strokes can be classified as deep effleurage or deep petrissage movements. Many have the misconception that to apply a deep stroke, you need to press harder with your hands or arms. My clients often think that I am stronger than I am, when actually I have learnt to use my body effectively to apply deeper work without effort. So again, I refer you to chapter 4: to work deeper and stronger, you must use your whole body to apply the stroke, not just your thumb or elbow, which can feel pokey and aggressive. Whenever you apply a deep stroke, you need to maintain control of the movement and work in cooperation with the tissue. Being too forceful and working too fast can cause tissue damage. Remember, the deeper you go, the slower you should go.

TIP The purposes of deep strokes:
- Separating tissue fascia
- Breaking down adhesions
- Realigning tissue
- Building strong mobile tissue

Control of any stroke should come from the legs (see chapter 4, Body Mechanics), with the arms well in front of you. In some instances, leaning your body over the movement will create more force, but it will also tend to squash the muscle into the bone, which can be uncomfortable.

At every opportunity it is important to reinforce your digits, especially if you have joints that are hypermobile. This will help to protect and prolong your career as a massage therapist. You can either assist your fingers by using other fingers or by applying the heel of your hand. The same can apply when using the thumb. Whichever part of your hand is making contact with your client should remain relaxed. The strength translates through the hand that is on top and the power of the stroke comes from your legs. See chapter 4 for further clarification.

To use an assisted thumb in this manner, place your thumb into the groove of the other hand, then turn over the hand and place it on the client. The top hand is where the power comes from and the bottom hand that is making contact with the client's skin is relaxed. If the bottom hand stiffens up the thumb will feel knifelike; make it easy on yourself and keep it soft.

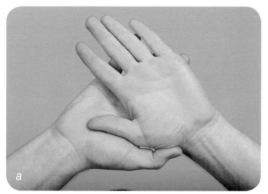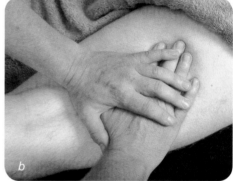

*(a)*Assisted thumbs and *(b)* placement of assisted thumbs on a client.

The key to this being an easy and effective stroke is to keep your elbow tucked into your hip, and as you move forward the strength will be generated from your hip. Therefore, if you find your arm has lost contact with your body, then the effort of the stroke has moved into your arm and away from your hip. Tucking the elbow into the hip makes the stroke easy, while losing contact puts stress onto your arms, shoulder and back. This can be a very strong stroke, so remember to go slower and check with your client to determine what is comfortable for him.

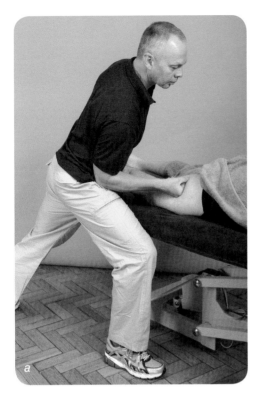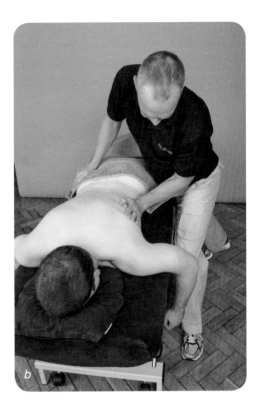

(a) Fist and (b) heel of hand.

Whether using your fist or the heel of your hand, make sure to position your body so that you are at a 45 degree angle, thus encouraging the tissue to move along the bone rather than pressing into it.

CLIENT TALK

When using a tucked arm stroke, there is a tendency for therapists to over shoot their position. Their knees go past the end of their foot, putting a stress on their knees. They are also prone to allow the arm to come away from their body, which in turn decreases the consistency and puts stress into their shoulder and arm. It is better to move and reposition yourself in order to finish the massage rather than keeping your feet stuck to the ground.

The heel of the hand is the focal point for transmitting the pressure to the tissue without stressing the digits. Ensure your fingers are relaxed and in contact with the tissue. Keep them soft rather than stiff. The fingers can be purposeful within the movement, but should follow rather than lead the heel of the hand. The heel of the hand in this instance is the leader. To finish the stroke all the way up the length of the leg muscle, you must make sure that your fingers are pointing away and do not end up in places they shouldn't. Keep your arms in a circular fashion so that your fingers are automatically pointing in the right direction, no matter which line of the leg you are working on.

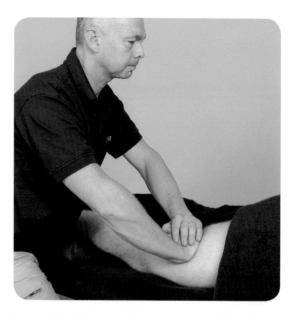

Longitudinal deep stroke using assisted hands.

Whenever you choose to use the elbow, be sure the depth of the muscle can handle the precision and force that it can offer. At first, students always comment that they cannot feel anything, but as you use your elbow more, your sensitivity will increase. Therefore, initially you should use it with caution so as to maintain a strong yet soft approach. A quick check to maintain a noninvasive approach is to make sure that your hand and wrist are relaxed; this will translate through the whole of the arm and help to prevent any unwanted force. Lower yourself by taking a wider stance in order to maintain the alignment of your torso to feet. This will protect your back and you will be able to apply a suitably deep stroke without pressing directly into the bone. For added protection and control you can place the other hand around the elbow using the space between the thumb and forefinger.

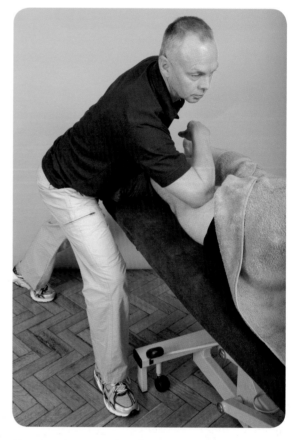

Deep stroke using the elbow.

CLIENT TALK

A simple way to check to see if your arm is relaxed is to check what your hand and wrist are doing. Visualize how supple yet strong a swan's movement is. Keep your wrist soft in the shape of a swan's neck and head; this will encourage a deep but smooth movement through the tissue.

Using the forearm is useful on most parts of the body, but care needs to be taken when applying this technique to the back. You need to be mindful of any bony prominences, in particular the spine. Make sure you are using the soft tissue portion of your forearm and avoid any pressure over the vertebrae. When you get up to the area of the scapulae, change the direction of your arm to avoid direct pressure over the bone. When using your forearm on the torso, use the bulky part of the muscle of your forearm to apply this stroke. Keep your arm ahead of you to push the tissue rather than be in line with the movement and thereby compressing the muscles into the ribs. The angle of your arm is such that the hand is quite a bit lower than the elbow; this will encourage the elbow to raise and prevent you from pressing down into the bony prominences of the spine.

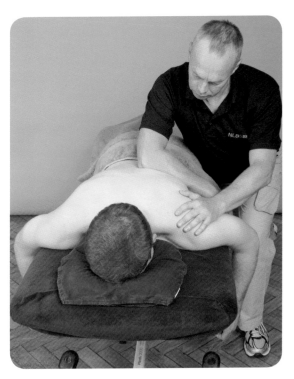

Deep stroke using the forearm.

There are two points that you need to consider when working directly over a specific area. First, consider if you are squashing the tissue into the bone and causing any discomfort to your client. Second, the angle at which you are working through your wrist must be considered. The closer it is to a 90 degree angle, the more stress it will put on the joint. While sometimes this might appear to be necessary to work in this position, it is not advisable to make it common practice. Place yourself over your extended arm. In this position it is

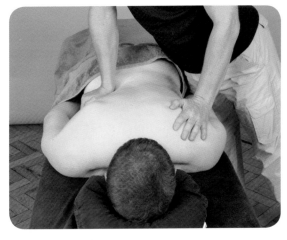

Working directly over tissue.

usually the weight of your body falling through the movement towards the floor that is sufficient to generate the power. Be mindful of the structures underneath your hands and check that your client is not suffering any undue stress.

Using an outstretched arm, place it onto the opposite side of the body from where you are working. It is important to generate the movement from the hips at arms length, this will create a smooth, deep or superficial stroke with ease. You can modify it to be either specific or broad by either flattening the hand or reinforcing the fingers as needed. It can be used on the torso, shoulders, legs and hip area and feels great. Placing one hand over the other, take the shape of the body part you are working with, extend the arms, allow the shoulders to relax, and using a wide asymmetrical stance, pull back using the hips. This is a time it is a requirement to allow the hips to lead as if you were going to sit on a chair. This technique can be applied to the whole of the torso as well.

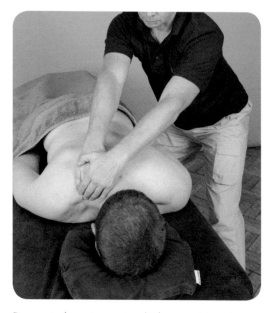

Deep stroke using extended arms. Note how the hips are pulling back.

TIP If the muscle flicks at the end of the movement on the shoulder, slow down the speed and lighten the pressure at the end of the stroke.

Vibration

Conventionally, the application of vibration involves quick movements to match the rate of nerve impulses to the muscles. Because that rate is too fast for you to reproduce without increasing the risk of injury to joints and other structures (including your own), it is best to use a rhythmical rate that suits you and the structures' ability to receive. Vibration can be used in an event situation or during a massage session. It assists in relaxing or stimulating the muscles, depending on the strength and vigour of the application. It can be applied superficially or deeply, gently or strongly. Whenever it is a more vigorous movement, the joints must be protected. If you need to get a better grip, especially if you are using lotion, work through a towel.

TIP The purposes of vibration:

- Dry technique
- Decreasing muscle hypertonicity
- Relaxing
- Stimulating

It is important to stay relaxed while applying vibration movements. Any tension you have will translate into the technique and make your movements feel jerky and stiff. The massage should feel like a flowing, rhythmical movement for both you and your client.

With the client in a prone position, bend his leg and place your hand on his heel. In this position you can either move the tissue with one of your hands while holding the client's heel or move the leg slightly back and forth using the hand on the heel in a rhythmical fashion. The key to applying this technique in this position is not to force the muscle to move, but to encourage it to move easily from side to side.

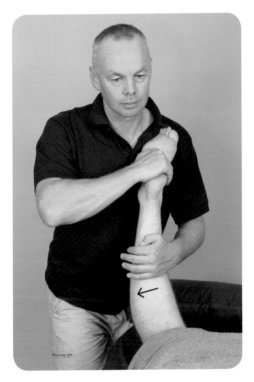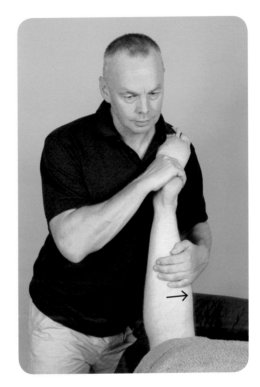

Vibration demonstrated on a bent leg.

CLIENT TALK

In all vibration movement techniques there needs to be a certain amount of depth and control while maintaining a relaxed movement. You can either apply it lightly or deeply, the main point is to control the movement and keep it within a limited area. It is a bit like whooshing water back and forth in a vase; it looks easy yet it is controlled. Your hands become the structure that prevents the tissue from going any further thus allowing the tissue to relax as it is able to sense it is in a controlled environment.

Place the palm of your hand on the larger muscle groups of the back and shake either up and down or across (or, my preference, in a circular fashion). You can apply this technique either lightly on the superficial tissue, or deeply by gathering up the layers. The same principle applies as in other techniques: the deeper you go, the slower your movement should be.

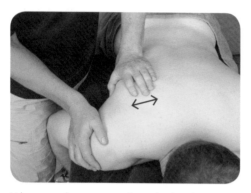
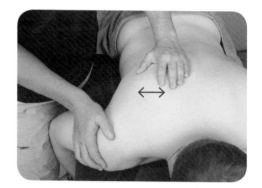

Vibration demonstrated on the back.

When working on the arm, be aware of the effects this movement will have on the elbow joint. Place your hands on either side of the arm and rotate the tissue around from front to back while moving down the arm. It is a bit like rubbing silly putty in your hands to make a long ropey structure. Do not over-rotate. Also, if there are any sounds or sensations that would indicate that the joint is being stressed, either change the rate and depth of application or choose another technique.

TIP If you have problems getting down on to your knees, this is not the position for you. Make sure you are in a comfortable and stable position.

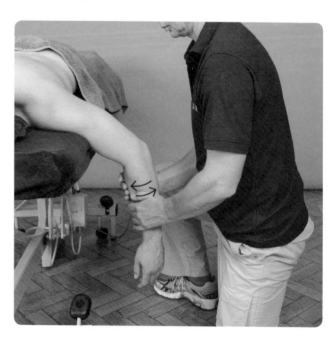

Vibration demonstrated on the arm.

Tapotement

Tapotement comes from the French word *tapoter*, which means 'to rap, drum or pat'. A good way to think of it is to associate it with playing the drums. As with drums, this technique requires both coordination and rhythm. It can be applied softly or heavily, quickly or slowly, depending on your purpose. It is another dry technique that requires no lubrication. It can be used in a number of circumstances such as event work, but also for clients who have breathing difficulties such as those with cystic fibrosis or asthma. In these circumstances tapotement helps to disperse any accumulation of fluids in the chest.

TIP The purposes of tapotement:

- Relaxing
- Stimulating
- Enhancing muscle tone
- Stimulating skin
- Stimulating muscle contraction
- Dry technique
- Breaking up fluid congestion in the lungs
- Stimulating sensory receptors

The key to applying this technique is maintaining an upright posture and relaxed arms. By keeping soft, bent legs and your arms at 90 degrees, you can control the force and be as strong or as gentle as needed. The various tapotement methods are suitable for different situations. For instance, when you need a more diffuse application of the technique, cupping is preferable.

When using tapotement, avoid striking over any bony prominences such as the vertebrae. Be cautious when working over the kidney area and when working around the lower back in clients who are in a sensitive part of their menstrual cycle. Another sensitive area to be aware of is the back of the knees. Keep moving from one place to another, avoid striking the same spot repeatedly, try to be methodical and do not space your contact areas too far apart.

The following are a few examples of tapotement techniques. Not everyone finds all of these techniques easy; choose the ones that suit you and practise the others over time.

HACKING   Hacking is applied using the medial border of your hands, keeping your fingers and wrists soft, and allowing your fingers to strike the tissue. If the sound is solid, then your fingers are too rigid. Try relaxing them a bit more so that you hear a quick succession of sounds.

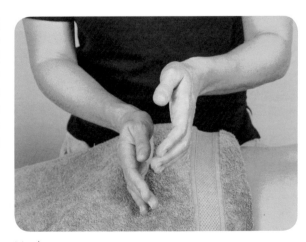

Hacking.

PRAYER   The key to this technique is to keep the elbows out, the heels of the hands pressed together and the fingers relaxed. As in hacking, the sound should be rhythmical rather than a solid thump.

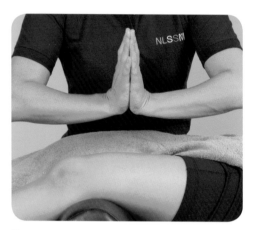 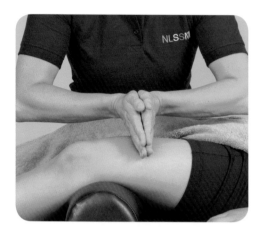

Prayer.

CUPPING   To form the shape of a cup, think of putting both hands together as if trying to fill them up with water; then separate them and turn them over so they are facedown, keeping this shape. Maintain the shape without being too rigid. You should be able to produce a hollow sound, not a slapping one.

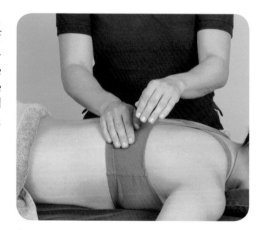

Cupping.

PUFFER   To perform the puffer technique, adopt the cupping position with your hands and then fold both hands on top of each other creating a structure that resembles a pod. The idea is to maintain this space when making contact and to allow some slight softening of the hands without collapsing them entirely. The sound should be as if air has escaped from between the hands. It can be difficult to get the right sound and control of the hands. Typical mistakes are allowing the hands to collapse too much when making contact, being too stiff or letting the hands separate.

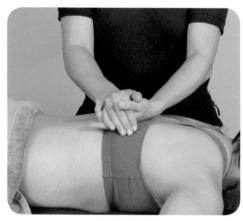

Puffer.

TAPPING Tapping is the lightest of all the tapotement strokes. It does not have a sound other than a light tapping from the fingertips.

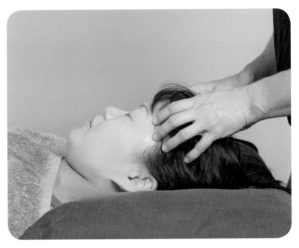

Tapping.

Friction

One of the primary purposes of friction is to break down fascial adhesions and scar tissue and to stimulate movement in tissue that has become stuck together. Friction encourages the separation and stretching of the tissue through the application of superficial, deep and precise strokes. It also separates the tissue of the muscle. This increases circulation to and movement in the area and promotes strong, mobile tissue, thus restoring function. Cautions and contraindications include fragile skin, neighbouring infections, recent scar tissue and decreased sensation (e.g., diabetes).

TIP The purposes of friction:

- Loosening tight tissues
- Breaking down adhesions and scar tissue
- Building strong, mobile tissue
- Realigning tissues
- Encouraging optimal repair of soft tissue
- Normalising injured tissues

In its classical sense, *friction* means to rub two surfaces together to create heat. This implies that the action is brisk. Friction can be used quickly when applied superficially, but it needs to be modified when working deeply. Slowing the speed down, allowing the tissue to 'melt' under the pressure and moving it thoughtfully will evoke a more meaningful change.

Thumbs, fingers, knuckles and elbows are the usual tools of choice. If you have bendy thumbs, avoid using them because doing so may stress your joints and instead choose a more comfortable approach (e.g., supported thumbs or digits). To test whether your thumb hyperextends, simply point your thumb up as if to signal everything is OK; if it bends backwards, use an alternative method. If your thumb resembles the right one (see the photo on page 62) that has a greater curvature to it then it is recommended you avoid using your thumb as much as possible. There will be a greater risk of injury to the joint because it will not be able to keep up with the demands placed on it. I would therefore suggest that right from the start of your career you adopt alternative methods in which to apply your deeper and more specific strokes.

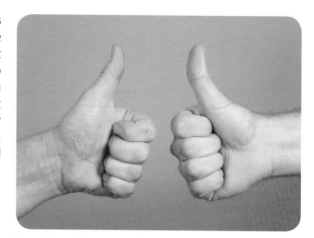

Normal and hyperextended thumbs.

TIP Minimise the use of a single thumb as a tool especially if it bends back beyond a straight line when extended. A single thumb is best used for very specific work and on muscles that are not large but that you need to go deeply into to get to the area you want to work on. A better option is to use a reinforced thumb, which will allow you to pinpoint a specific area without any tension or strain to your joints.

To use an assisted thumb technique, place one hand on the client's body with the thumb pointing out; this hand and the thumb remain passive, which means they carry no tension. Then place the other hand on top, using the groove of the upper hand to secure the thumb. The pressure of the movement comes from the top hand, and the power should be directed from the legs. If you want to be more specific, you can slightly bend the thumb under the hand if your joint can tolerate it. If your hand feels discomfort or stressed, either you are not applying the technique correctly or it is not suitable for you.

You can use either passive or active friction movements. A movement is passive when the client relaxes and you initiate the movement. With an active movement, the client is in control of the movement. The passive technique allows you to control the movement and be more precise. It also prevents uncontrolled movements that might cause damage to the tissue. By performing the technique passively prior to a client doing it actively, you can demonstrate what is expected. Asking a client to do an active movement gives you more hands to work with since you have freed up a hand by getting them to do the movement.

The depth of your friction technique is determined by which body part you are working on, your intent (superficially or deeply) and the tolerance of the client's tissue. The differences between working on the gluteus maximus and working on the chest are evidenced by the depth of the tissue. The larger the muscle and the deeper you need to work, the greater the importance is of applying the technique correctly and using the right tool. For larger muscles, you might choose to use your elbow, but in areas where the muscle is more shallow (e.g., on and around the scapula) you might choose assisted fingers. It is equally important to evaluate your client's pain tolerance and whether you are applying too much pressure. For a more in-depth discussion about pain, read the Pain Assessment section in chapter 9, Client Assessment.

In the same way as you apply deep strokes, you can apply friction using similar tools and follow the same principles of application. The main difference is that deep strokes are moving techniques that take you the length of the muscle or across it, while friction tends to be more about remaining in a particular spot to break down tough, hardened tissue. You might choose to apply it transversely, longitudinally or in a circular fashion, helping to soften it up and realign the fibres. You have a choice of using a variety of tools, as seen in the deep strokes section of this chapter. Whatever you choose, always remember to flush and relax the area with general techniques such as effleurage, petrissage or vibration.

Top 10 Tips for the Successful Application of Friction

1. Warm up the tissue first.
2. Place the client in a relaxed position.
3. Do not compress heavily into the bone.
4. Watch your speed; don't go too fast.
5. Get feedback from the client.
6. Use breathing techniques to help with relaxation.
7. Do not overwork the area.
8. Combine with flushing techniques.
9. Use ice cube therapy (optional).
10. Watch your own technique; do not overstress your digits.

Table 5.1   Summary of Massage Techniques

Stroke	Purposes	Effects	Specific contraindications
Effleurage	<ul><li>Warms the tissue</li><li>Introduces your touch</li><li>Relaxes the client</li><li>Spreads lotion</li><li>Allows you to palpate and assess tissue</li><li>Flushes</li><li>Is a connecting technique</li></ul>	<ul><li>Enhances arterial, venous and lymphatic circulation</li><li>Increases cellular metabolism</li><li>Decreases muscular tension</li><li>Decreases pain</li><li>Decreases ischemia</li></ul>	
Petrissage	<ul><li>Relaxes muscles and general tension</li><li>Provides a deeper stroke</li><li>Separates tissue (e.g., fascial adhesions, scar tissue)</li></ul>	<ul><li>Increases circulation</li><li>Stimulates sebaceous gland activity, softens skin</li><li>Relieves pain</li></ul>	

»continued

Table 5.1 »continued

Stroke	Purposes	Effects	Specific contraindications
Compression	■ Warms up, flushes and relaxes ■ Deactivates hypertonicity when using deeper strokes ■ Decreases muscle spasms ■ Can be used as a dry technique at events ■ Affects other tissue receptors	■ Increases circulation ■ Increases heat ■ Decreases pain	■ Joints that are loose ■ Excessive compression ■ Brittle bone disease (i.e., severe osteoporosis)
Deep strokes	■ Separate tissue, fascia ■ Break down adhesions ■ Realign tissue ■ Promote strong, mobile tissue	■ Increases circulation ■ Increases movement	
Vibration	■ Warms up ■ Stimulates the muscle ■ Relaxes the client ■ Can be used as a dry technique at events ■ Decreases muscle hypertonicity	■ Increases temperature of tissue ■ Decreases pain sensitivity ■ Increases circulation	■ Excessive vibration ■ Brittle bone disease (i.e., severe osteoporosis) ■ Excessive movement to the joint ■ Loose joints as a result of pregnancy or hypermobility
Tapotement	■ Stimulates sensory receptors ■ Can be used as a warm-up (light application) ■ Relaxes the client ■ Can be used as a dry technique at events ■ Enhances muscle tone ■ Breaks up fluid congestion in lungs ■ Stimulates muscle contraction	■ Increases circulation	■ Muscle spasm or cramping ■ Atrophied muscles ■ Over bony areas ■ Pregnancy ■ No *heavy* tapotement over the kidneys and lower back ■ Severe osteoporosis
Friction	■ Loosens tight tissues ■ Breaks down fascial adhesions and scar tissue ■ Realigns tissue and builds strong connections ■ Encourages optimal repair and normalisation of injured tissues	■ Increases circulation ■ Increases the temperature of tissues	■ Haematoma ■ Myositis ossificans (calcifications) ■ Acute injury ■ Fragile skin ■ Neighbouring infections ■ Recent scar tissue ■ Decreased sensation

Closing Remarks

All the techniques in this chapter constitute a good foundation, but by no means are they limited in their application method or style. As you gain experience, you will develop your own style, try various approaches, vary your techniques or even combine them. I have learnt so much from watching others, playing around with what I have and receiving massage. As a result, I have developed my own unique approach, as will you. As long as your technique is safe, feels good and is effective, you have all the right components to deliver a massage that clients will return for.

Quick Questions

1. Why should you start your massage strokes superficially?
2. Which techniques can be used as initial warm-up techniques?
3. What are four contraindications and cautions you need to consider when using friction?
4. What must you consider before applying tapotement?
5. To go deeper, you must go_____.

PART III

Applying Sports Massage

People often have a preconception that there are only two positions in massage, prone "and" supine. Unlike conventional massage therapists, however, sports massage therapists frequently change their clients' positions to access muscles more effectively. Therefore, at the onset of your training you need to learn how to be comfortable moving a client around. I would suggest that you revisit chapters 4 and 5, "Body Mechanics" and "Massage Techniques" while working through this part since they will help reinforce a comfortable and powerful posture while working in each of these positions.

The chapters in this part address advanced working positions in prone, supine, side-lying and sitting positions. You will learn how to use the couch effectively to apply a variety of strokes. The focus is on the importance of your posture and client management. This will lay the groundwork for more advanced soft tissue techniques. The photos demonstrate ideas and help you to visualise the written information, but by no means are they intended to replace practical instruction from a tutor. A tutor can share knowledge and experience and help you see the need to make adjustments in both your technique and your client's position that you might not be aware of.

Each chapter addresses positioning your client, positioning yourself and applying safety features for both of you. Tip boxes make suggestions about how to self-check, which will reinforce your understanding of safe and effective positioning. As much as possible the chapters offer full descriptions of each position and technique, but remember that there is room to develop your own approach as well. If at any time you do not feel comfortable performing a technique, revisit what you are doing and make adjustments until it feels natural and does not place any stress on you.

Sports Massage for Prone Positions

Prone is a term that is used to describe a person who is either lying facedown on a massage couch or facing into an on-site massage chair. In most forms of massage prone is considered the primary client position, but in sports massage it is one of many. The prone position is useful for accessing the posterior muscles and limbs of the body. It provides easy access to most areas of the body, but its limitations also need to be considered. For instance, in this position you are working downwards into the tissue, which at times may not be the best choice because of the depth or placement of the targeted muscle. Always keep in mind all other possibilities and choose the one best suited for the circumstance. For the most part, the prone position is easy for clients to get into and often helps them relax and become quiet.

TIP To keep yourself adaptable and responsive to your clients, try to avoid always starting a massage with the client in a prone position. Consider what other choices are available and choose the best position for the needs of your client and the purpose of the treatment rather than getting into a habit or routine of placing a client facedown to start.

When positioning a client, make sure she is comfortable and her joints are protected. Place pillows or cushions in such a way as to support and give ease to limbs. Placement can include under the ankles, hips, chest or shoulders depending on the needs of the client.

- Placing support under the ankles helps to prevent excessive plantar flexion of the foot. Check to see that the cushion is away from the knees and supporting the whole of the foot. Make sure the cushion is soft enough to allow movement when you place pressure on the limb.
- If there is any history or indications of lower back problems, place a pillow under the pelvis and lower back.

- Clients with large breasts might find it more comfortable to have a pillow under the ribs.

- To support protracted shoulders, place a couple of small cushions or towels underneath.

- If your couch's face hole is uncomfortable or hard, a face cushion can solve this problem.

On the following pages are more advanced instructions for applying sports massage techniques to various areas of the body while your client is in a prone position. Choose techniques that are appropriate for these areas; for instance, tapotement on the neck is not a good choice, but gentle transverse effleurage on either side of the cervical spine is.

TIP Seek feedback from your clients to make sure they are feeling supported and comfortable. Many clients will not tell you that they are uncomfortable unless prompted.

It is important when working on the neck to determine whether the client has any conditions that would prohibit work in this area. It is a sensitive part of the body and needs to be approached with caution. Be mindful of your pressure, keep it light and work slowly, gradually going deeper. Check with your client for any signs of discomfort.

Neck Massage Technique 1

Place your hands one on top of the other using your fingertips on either side of the spine of the neck, evenly applying effleurage strokes away from the cervical spinous process and moving transversely across the muscles. An alternative stroke is working either direction longitudinally towards the occipital bone of the head or towards the shoulder.

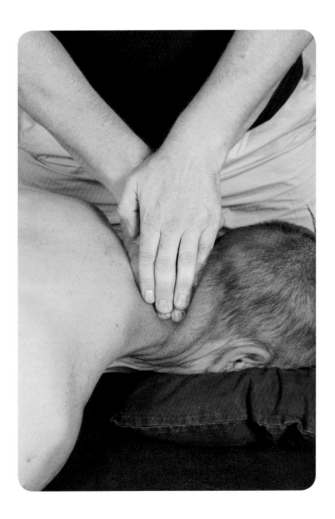

Shoulder Massage Technique 1

To apply a deep stroke across the anterior upper trapezius, place the heel of the hand on the inside of the shoulder. Place the other hand on the opposite shoulder to help you stabilize the client and to square your hips to face the direction you are moving. Move away from the neck, avoiding any deep pressure on the bony structures of the shoulder. This stroke will help lengthen the shoulders away from the neck.

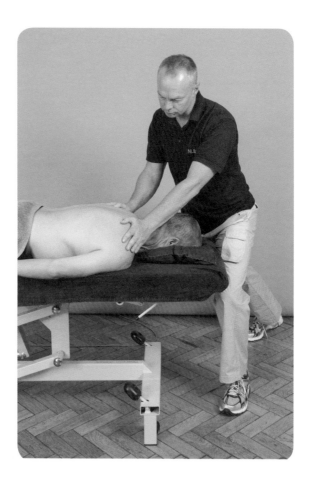

Shoulder Massage Technique 2

Standing on one leg, place your knee that is closer to the top of the client's head onto the couch above the client's shoulder. Keep your hips and torso squared onto the movement, maintaining an upright posture. Place your hands on the client's opposite shoulder, working across the couch. Using a rhythmical petrissage action, pick up and lift the tissue. By maintaining a circle with your arms (keep the elbows out), you will get a much more fluid and stronger movement.

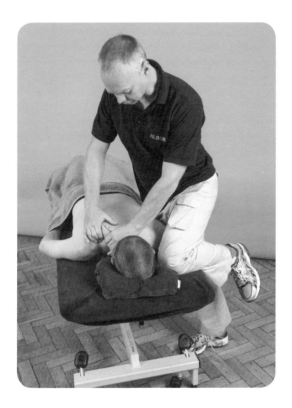

TIP If you find you are having to hitch up your hips to get your leg up on the couch, lower the couch height. This lower position may actually be the correct height for you. Stepping onto a platform or box is never a safe way to work.

CLIENT TALK

Throughout all the chapters, keep in mind to use a combination of strokes and techniques to maintain a flow as you make your transitions from one stroke to another. You will develop your own style, taking into consideration how you like to move around the couch and what techniques you favour, but always think about the continuity of your movements and how they are connected to each other. It helps to keep your hands on the client as much as possible to maintain that continuous flow.

Shoulder Massage Technique 3

Partially sit on the couch lifting one leg off the floor but using the other to anchor your position by pushing your foot down into the floor. Place the client's arm over your leg. Ensure that your posture is upright while applying the various massage moves. This position gives you access to the whole of the shoulder, anterior and posterior, as well as the arm.

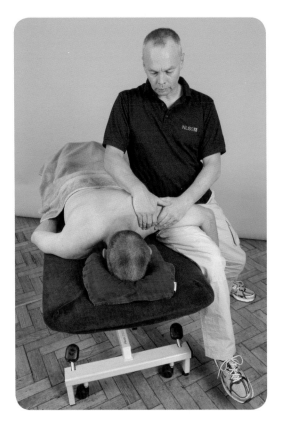

TIP This is an excellent opportunity to work on the anterior of the shoulder while a client is prone. This is often the area that needs to be released with clients that have protracted shoulders. Elongating the muscles in the front allows the shoulders to open up and relax. I often warm up the muscles in this position before I turn the client over to do some more specific work.

Shoulder Massage Technique 4

Massaging around the scapula can at times be difficult because of the tendency for the tissue to be stretched in the prone position. If this is the case, try positioning your arm underneath the client's shoulder while standing and facing towards the client's upper body. Cup the top of the shoulder joint in your hand. Lift the shoulder by pressing your elbow into the couch while lifting the heel of your hand. This should give some ease to the tissue so that you can work on the surrounding muscles. This position allows you to do a multitude of techniques, such as deep, long strokes under and around the scapula, and also gives you the opportunity to do some mild stretching and mobilisation work.

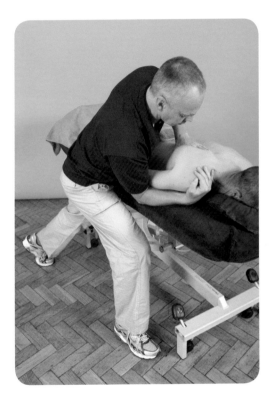

TIP Maintaining a flat back and using your legs to support your stance will make it much easier to lift the client's shoulder. If you have a slouched posture, you will have difficulty raising the client's shoulder because you will be using your upper body to do the mechanics of the lift rather than taking advantage of sinking your hips to lever up the client's shoulder.

Torso Massage Technique 1

To work across the client onto the opposite side of the torso, adopt a wide side stance position, press your thighs into the couch and use it as an anchor as you gather the tissue in towards yourself. Using the couch in this manner allows you to increase the strength of your stroke yet also helps to stabilise your posture.

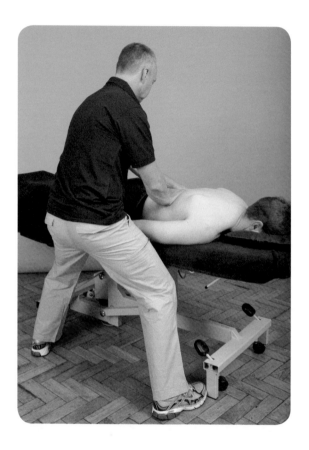

Torso Massage Technique 2

Using an asymmetrical stance, place the hands on the rib area of the torso. Put one hand on top of the other and keep the hand underneath relaxed and apply the pressure from the top hand. You can apply either a broad or specific, targeted stroke. If you want to get into the intercostal muscles between the ribs, use an assisted hand/digit technique to apply specific pressure from a single digit. For a broader or more general stroke, apply pressure evenly across the hand and fingers.

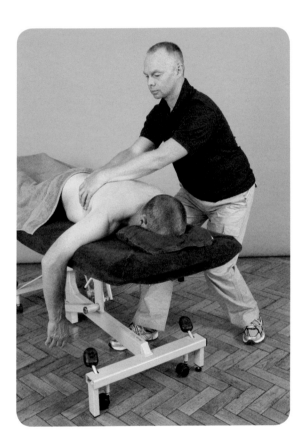

Pelvis Massage Technique 1

The pelvis can be massaged either through a towel or by direct contact from either side of the couch. Working from the opposite side of the couch is only suitable if your stature allows you to do this comfortably. If you feel any stress in your lower back from having to reach over too far, it is not a position of choice for you.

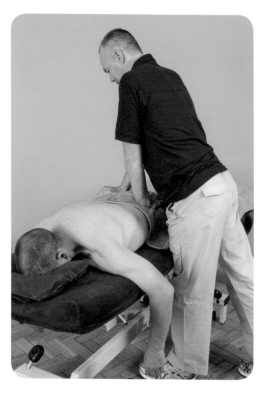
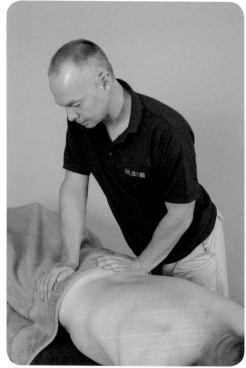

Pelvis Massage Technique 2

Position yourself on the same side of the couch that you want to work on. It is best to use the heel of your hand to massage the bulk of the gluteal muscles as these are generally strong and deep muscles. Try to minimize the use of your digits and save them for more specific work. Apply your strokes at a 45-degree angle to ensure that you lift the tissue away, rather than squishing it into the bone; this also helps to protect your wrists. Movements can be applied in all directions—transverse, longitudinal and circular.

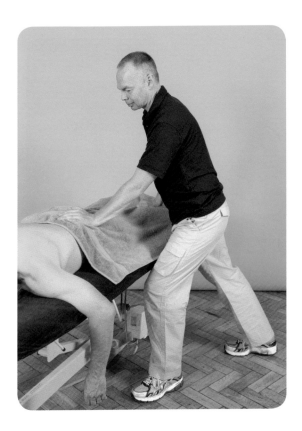

TIP When changing the direction of your massage stroke (e.g., from working towards the head to working towards the legs), make sure your stance is square onto the direction of the stroke. This change of direction is initiated by placing your foot behind the movement and maintaining a broad stance. Because the muscles of the pelvis can be very strong, to get the desired depth you need to generate your strength from your base, which is your foot.

Leg Massage Technique 1

When the natural position of the client's leg is too externally rotated to allow you access to the muscles at the side of the leg, use one hand to control the leg's direction by placing one hand on the leg and moving it into the position that opens up the area. This will enable you to apply your strokes with the other hand to the whole of the leg. A word of caution: When moving up the leg towards the torso, lighten up on the depth of your stroke when passing behind the knee because of the sensitive structures located there.

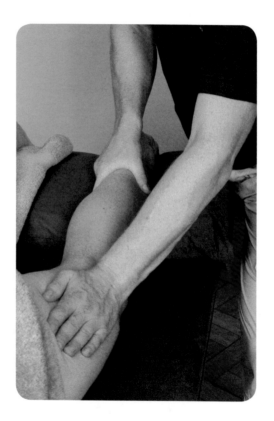

Leg Massage Technique 2

Before sitting on the couch, remove the cushion or pillow from the side of the couch. Assume a stable position by bending the leg closer to the middle of the couch and extending the other leg to the floor to stabilise your position. Always keep one foot in contact with the floor to ensure your safety and help you maintain an upright posture. Bend the client's leg and rest it on your shoulder. This position is only suitable if you and your client are a similar size; if you are larger than your client, you will end up having to slouch to get the client's foot onto your shoulder. This position allows the tissues to drop away from the skeletal structure making it easier to access some of the deeper muscles of the calf such as the soleus.

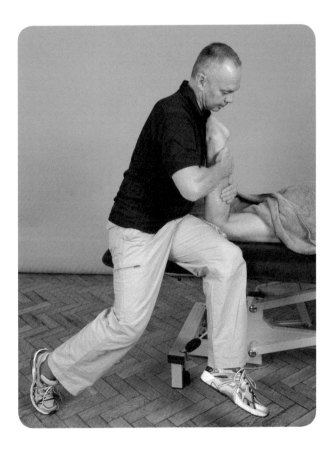

Leg Massage Technique 3

Use the couch to its fullest advantage while standing by placing your inside leg onto the couch without hitching up your hip. Place the lower leg of your client onto your thigh. This position allows you to remain upright while working deeper into the tissue and is also useful when applying more advanced techniques such as soft tissue release.

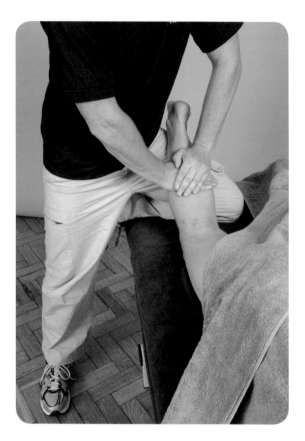

TIP Make sure a button or zipper on your clothing or a wallet in your pocket does not aggravate your client's skin. You can place a towel on your leg if you are wearing shorts or you do not want lotion on your clothing.

Leg Massage Technique 4

Standing on the opposite side of the couch can be a useful position from which to apply massage strokes to the leg. This position is effective for a number of strokes, but it is particularly effective for wringing, lifting, or gathering movements. A word of caution is needed, though: If your stature does not allow you to do this without reaching over and putting stress on your back, then this position is not for you.

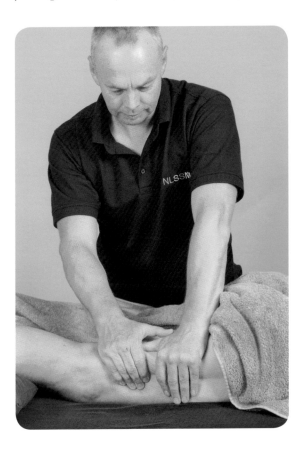

Foot Massage Technique 1

In a standing position, place one leg on the couch and your client's foot on your outer thigh; this allows you to face the direction of the foot. This is a comfortable position for both you and your client, and it helps keep the foot stable so you can apply deeper and more specific strokes to the area. The use of fingers and thumbs is more appropriate here because the surface area is very small. Using the heel of the hand in a flushing action is effective, and it feels great for the client. The direction of your stroke is not limited because it will not interfere with the circulatory system.

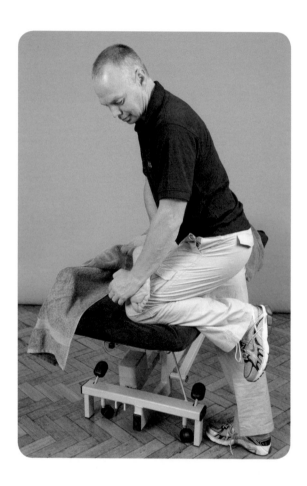

On-site massage can stand alone or be adapted to a variety of situations. It involves the use of a very mobile piece of equipment that does not take up much room, and you can do all your work applying dry techniques through clothing. You can simply take what you have learnt as a sport massage therapist and adapt it to the chair. Other forms of on-site chair massage incorporate other massage modalities, such as acupressure, Swedish massage, and shiatsu. You can take further training to develop those methods or use them in applying sport massage. Following are examples of adapting a typical couch technique to the chair.

On-Site Chair Technique 1

In applying a general massage technique at this angle, you need to change the position of your arms and the direction of your stroke. The arms are still extended away from you and the power is still coming from your legs, but the movement is more in and up than down and along.

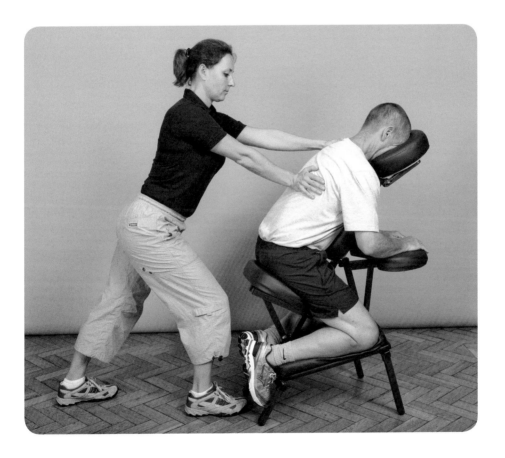

On-Site Chair Technique 2

In the same manner as you would do a deep stroke using a straight arm position, place yourself diagonally from the opposite side and pull slowly around the top of the shoulder using your hips to create the movement and keeping your arms extended but relaxed. If the tissue flips underneath your hands, try going more slowly.

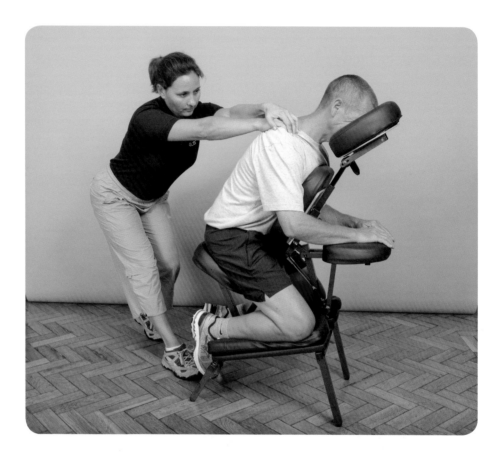

Quick Questions

1. What are the advantages to using a seated position on the couch to work on the shoulders?
2. How many times was the phrase 'maintain an upright posture' mentioned in this chapter?
3. When placing a client's leg on your thigh, what must you be aware of?
4. Why is it appropriate to use thumbs and digits on the feet and not on the gluteus maximus?
5. In which area of the body do you need to exercise greater caution?

7

Sports Massage for Supine Positions

Supine is a term used to describe a person lying on his back, facing up. Typically, in this position the arms, legs and a bit of the chest and neck are massaged. An area often neglected is the torso (the abdominal region and chest). This seems a bit odd considering that the muscles in this area play an integral part in movement and breathing. If your client has postural imbalances, then working the torso area is a must to rebalance tensions and give ease to the muscles posteriorly. The list of reasons to give more attention to massaging the whole of the torso is long. If your course of instruction does not address the specifics of abdominal massage, I recommend looking into doing a continuing professional development course to obtain the necessary skills to work in this area.

TIP When a client is in a supine position, the chest, abdominal and pelvic regions require a sensitive approach. When working in these areas, do not focus your gaze on what you are doing, but allow your hands to see and take your gaze elsewhere. Work through a towel as much as possible, and apply your strokes in a confident manner. Clients will pick up any nervousness in you, which will create the same feeling in them.

To ensure that your client is comfortable and well supported, place pillows under her head and knees to support the joints and give ease to the back.

On the following pages are more advanced instructions for a variety of sports massage techniques that you can use while your client is in the supine position. Be sure you have mastered the basic massage techniques (covered in chapters 4 and 5) before progressing to these more advanced techniques.

You need to take special care when working on the neck. A sensitive approach is essential. To gain your client's trust, make sure you feel confident when she places her head in your hands. Start by making sure that your legs give you the necessary wide base, your shoulders are relaxed, your arms are straight and the couch is at the right height to allow you to do this comfortably.

Neck Massage Technique 1

Establishing your posture first is the key to this technique. Place one leg behind in a comfortable long stance; this will allow you to move slightly backwards when performing the stroke. Your shoulders should be away from your ears, your arms should be straight and your palms up. Place one hand under the client's head, while the other starts the stroke at the base of the neck near the shoulders. With palms facing up, smoothly bring the hand farther from you towards the base of the skull. The other hand should support the head until the moving hand has reached the top of the neck. Then switch hands; the active hand now takes the supportive role while the other one starts the process over again on the opposite side.

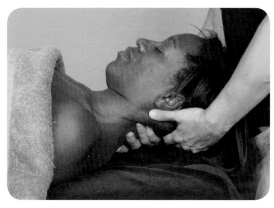

These next two photos show you what your hands should look like while completing this technique. Note that you would not place your client in this position to do this stroke; these photos are simply to illustrate how your hands are placed.

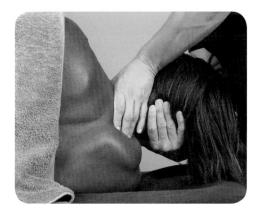
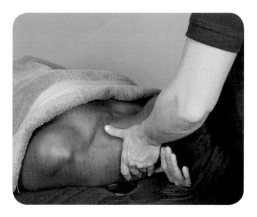

TIP Get feedback from your client. If it feels as though she is holding her head up for you, then reevaluate your position and how comfortable you are. You must perform this process smoothly to get the results you want. The three key points are to move from your legs; maintain straight arms; and relax, or drop, your shoulders.

Neck Massage Technique 2

Place both legs in a wide side stance (the second position in ballet if you can relate to that). Cup the base of the client's head with one hand with a straight arm and relaxed shoulders. Gently turn the head slightly away from the side you are applying the stroke to. In other words, if you plan to use your right arm along the right side of the client's neck, turn the client's head to the left as you are doing this. It is important to keep the client's head in a stable and supported position throughout.

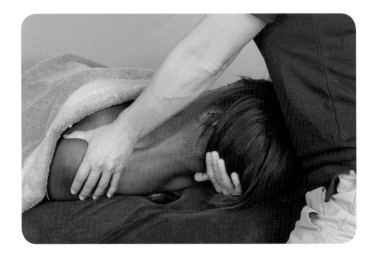

When working on the chest in the supine position, make sure the towel is placed in such a way as to maintain privacy whether your client is male or female. Avoid looking down at the area you are working on because this is less invasive to your client. As you gain experience, your hands will get better at being able to sense where you are.

Chest Massage Technique 1

Place one hand on top of the other and work across the chest, below the clavicle, from the midline to the shoulder using a long, gliding stroke. When altering the direction of your stroke, rather than turning from the upper torso, change the placement of your foot and keep your hips and shoulders squared onto the movement. If the area allows it (i.e., your hands are small enough), or there is a larger surface area in which to work, you can use the heel of your hand instead of the finger pads.

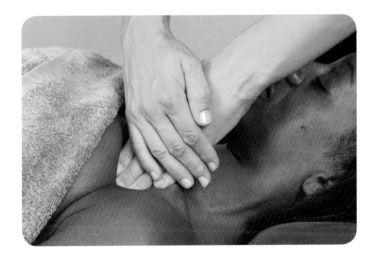

TIP Even when you do not have a lot of room in which to work, using both hands, one on top of the other, helps to keep your shoulders and body squared onto the area you are massaging and prevents you from inadvertently placing your unoccupied hand where it shouldn't be.

Shoulder and Arm Massage Technique 1

Place the client's bent arm into your abdomen. Your abdominal muscles become the anchor that allows you to control the movement so you can have both arms available to apply your techniques. This is a comfortable position for both you and your client, but it requires that your couch be at the right height and that your client's elbow be securely placed into your abdomen.

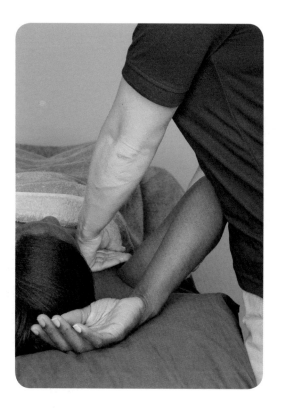

CLIENT TALK

This position is also good for easier access to the whole of the upper arm as well as a great many of the muscles of the shoulder girdle. You might also be able to access the edge of the subscapularis, normally a hard muscle to get to. If you can master controlling the client's arm with your torso, then you have two arms available to work with. On another note, be aware of the structures in this area, such as lymph nodes, as they can be quite sensitive to pressure.

Shoulder and Arm Massage Technique 2

Another option for working on the arms and shoulder area in the supine position is to hold your client's arm in your bent arm (the one closer to his midline). This technique is effortless if your shoulders are relaxed. Secure the arm close to your body, making sure you are using the supporting hand to control the movement. In order to help your client feel relaxed and supported, make sure the upper portion of the arm is resting on the couch.

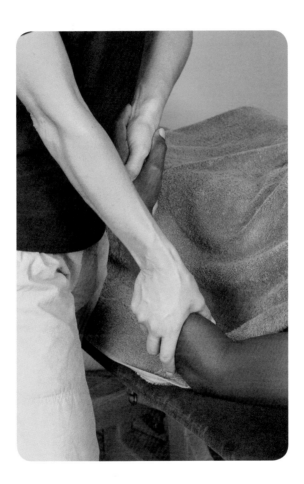

Abdominal work is an important part of sports massage treatment. It can be a specialty within massage, but for the purpose of this book we will address it only superficially. Abdominal massage has great benefits, especially when addressing postural and breathing issues.

Torso and Abdominal Muscles Massage Technique 1

Use a wide symmetrical stance and stand facing your client at their side by the abdominals. Begin to gently palpate the area, working in a clockwise manner to match the direction of the digestive system. You can apply a variety of strokes and methods of application (e.g., heel of hand, fists, knuckles) as long as you are careful not to be too invasive and to work with the structures beneath the more superficial layers.

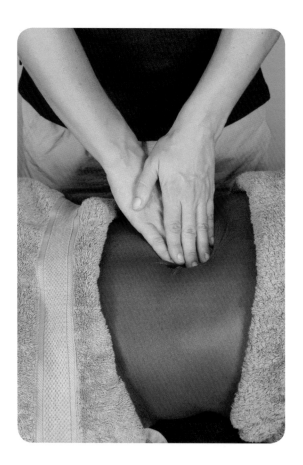

Torso and Abdominal Muscles Massage Technique 2

Depending on which part of the diaphragm you are massaging, you will need to adjust your position and the direction you are facing. Keep your foot and hips squared into the movement. It is easier to work across the table on the opposite side, but you can work on the same side if you apply the principle of creating a circle with your arms. To work along the diaphragm, place the edge of your hands along the border of the ribs and diaphragm. Monitor the depth by checking with your client about the level of comfort. Work with the rhythm of her breath to ease into the tissue and move slowly, adapting the depth of the stroke as you go. If you need to create more ease (i.e., decrease the tension) to the tissue, place one hand underneath the ribs around to the back and lift gently towards the midline.

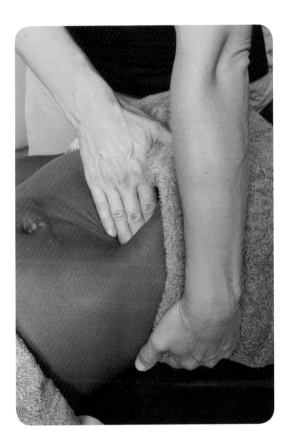

TIP To prevent any undue discomfort to your client, make sure your fingernails are short enough so they do not cut into the skin. You might also try to angle your fingers so they are not directly pushing into the ribs but working on their edge.

Torso and Abdominal Muscles Massage Technique 3

Using an asymmetrical stance with straight arms, place one hand on top of the other under the client's torso on the opposite side from your working position. Initially, direct the movement of your hands from your legs to lift up the tissue on the posterior portion of the torso and then allow your hips to pull back to create a transverse stroke. Follow around the curvature of the ribs up the lateral border of the torso using a flatter finger and hand placement to accommodate the lack of muscle mass.

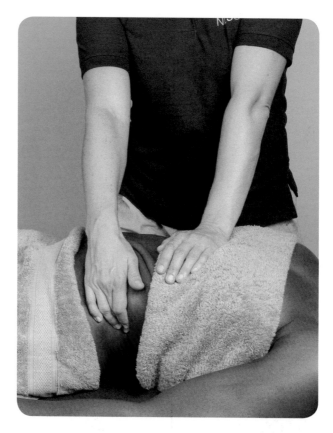

TIP If you want to do specific strokes between the ribs (into the intercostals), add a bit more pressure to one of the digits from the hand on top, keeping the bottom finger relaxed. Remember, the deeper and more precisely you work, the slower you need to go to minimise any discomfort.

The pelvis can be a sensitive area and there may be an issue with client modesty as well. Because clients need to feel comfortable and safe, ask their permission before beginning any work on the pelvis. I often work through a towel in this area.

Pelvis Massage Technique 1

Assume a comfortable position with your legs. You can use supported fingers, the heel of the hand, or whatever is comfortable for you and the client depending on the area you need to work on. The smaller the area, the smaller the tool. If you find the client's hip is moving too much, place one hand on the hip closer to you to help stabilise him. Be mindful of the bony prominences, and keep in mind that the tissue in this area can be quite sensitive or ticklish. Slower movements using the correct depth will minimise reactions such as twitching.

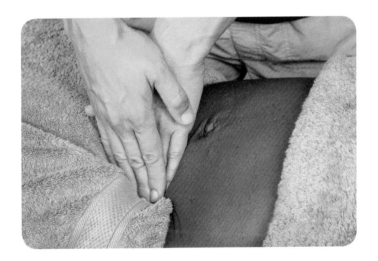

Thigh Massage Technique 1

Standing in either an asymmetrical or symmetrical position, reach across to the other side of the couch and place your hands on your client's outer thigh. You can use a deep cross friction technique by hooking your fingers into the tissue and using the legs to create the movement, or you can use petrissage, effleurage or broad transverse strokes up and down the whole of the thigh. As long as you are not struggling or placing any stress on your lower back as a result of reaching over to the other side of the couch (because of your size or your client's), then this is a suitable position to work from.

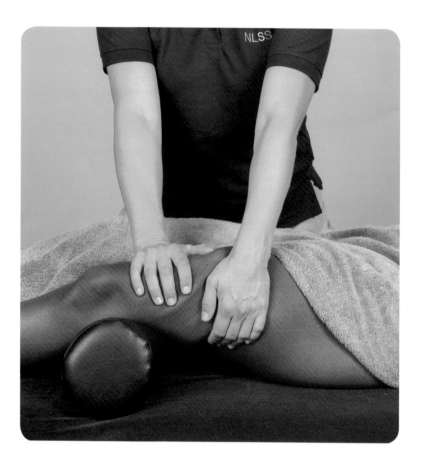

Thigh Massage Technique 2

Facing towards your client, place her foot on your shoulder with her knee bent at 90 degrees. To steady the limb, place one hand on the anterior lower portion of the thigh (not on the knee) and pull it towards your shoulder using enough strength to control the movement of the limb. Use the other hand to apply strokes to the posterior portion of the client's thigh, using your fist, the heel of your hand or your forearm.

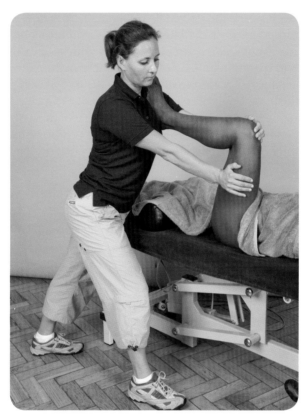

TIP It is very important that you maintain an upright posture, keeping your torso in alignment with your legs and using your legs to generate the movement and power.

CLIENT TALK

I find this position particularly useful when I am working with muscle imbalances between that of the pelvis and hamstrings. Also, there are situations where I will spend a suitable amount of time massaging the hamstrings and want to give it a rest before returning and doing a bit more work later but I do not want to keep turning my client over or I might be limited for time. Being able to move the body around to access various parts of the body regardless of what position the client is in is extremely useful and every effort should be made to make this a part of your normal routine.

Thigh Massage Technique 3

This technique should be used to apply an inner-thigh massage. Place your outer knee, or the one farther from the client's upper body, onto the couch, and then place the client's bent leg onto your thigh. Making sure that the majority of the client's thigh has no contact with you, turn your body to face directly towards the length of the client's leg. If you find yourself having to hitch your hip up to do this, lower the height of the couch. (If you are working at your optimal height, you should not have to do this.) Apply your massage strokes towards the pelvis. If you are using the heel of your hand, make sure your hand is turned towards the lateral side of the client's body and use the ulna border of your hand. Maintaining a circular position with your arms will reinforce the position. This helps to maintain an even depth for the length of the stroke.

Alternatively, you can change the direction of your stroke, working transversely across the adductors. In this case you will need to change your stance, reposition your leg, and turn to face the client's other leg. Again, make sure that most of the client's thigh is free of any contact with your thigh. This is an excellent position in which to use petrissage on the inner thigh, lifting up tissue from both the posterior and medial borders.

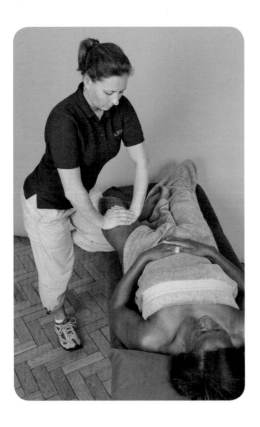
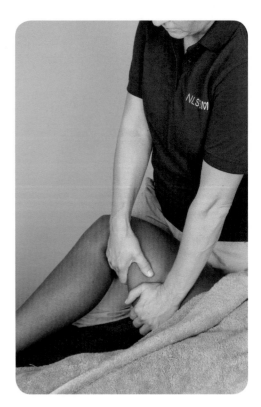

Leg Massage Technique 1

Bend your client's knee and sit on his foot. Sometimes a client will be a bit surprised by this and try to move his foot away from you. If this happens, explain that this helps to keep the leg from pushing forward. You can stabilise your own posture by extending your outside leg and pushing it into the floor. This position is useful for accessing both posterior and anterior calf muscles. In particular, the posterior muscles are able to hang loosely away from the skeletal structure making it easier to get to the deeper tissues.

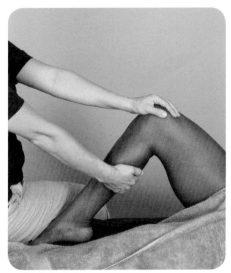 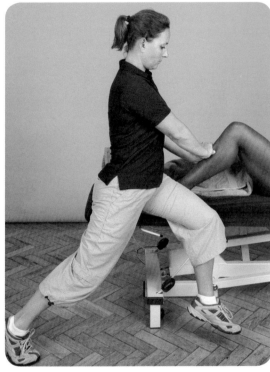

TIP It is easy to get the direction of the massage movement mixed up; simply make sure your movements are towards the knee (working with the circulatory system). In more advanced techniques this rule is not always followed.

Feet are often overlooked, yet they play an important role in the whole of the body movement patterns. They support us by translating the weight of our whole body into the ground. Understandably, they can get tired, stiff and overworked, yet more often than not very little attention is given to them. Mobilising, stretching and massaging the feet can have an enormous effect on the rest of the body. Some upper body injuries, for example, are attributed to foot dysfunction. I always tend to look at the body as one unit, rather than as small compartments that make up a whole. I evaluate the body globally to get a clear picture of how the various parts of the musculoskeletal system are interacting. If you elicit a tickling sensation when working on the feet, try applying a stronger, more confident stroke using the whole of your hand; this will usually solve the problem. Alternatively, you can work through a towel.

Foot Massage Technique 1

Use the heel of your hands to spread the tissue on the dorsal surface of the feet. Keep your arms long and allow your body weight to generate the force through the hands. You can either pull away from the legs or drop your weight over the stroke. This opening and separating action helps alleviate tension in the feet.

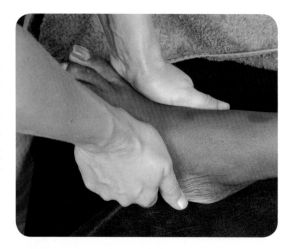

Even though the feet have a small surface area, you should still use your legs to lead your movements as much as possible to help maintain your posture. Taking a wide stance with one leg behind, bend your arm and press your elbow into your hip. Make a fist and use the flat part of your knuckles to push down the length of the foot, propelling the movement from your foot.

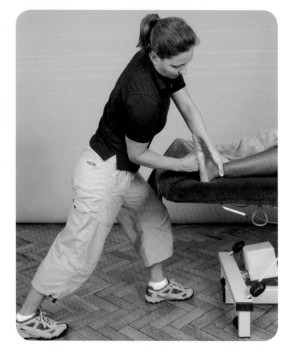

Quick Questions

1. When should you apply advanced techniques in the supine position?
2. Where should you place pillows to make your client comfortable and support the joints in a supine position?
3. In what direction should your strokes be to assist the digestive tract?
4. What can you do to make your clients more comfortable when working in sensitive areas?
5. What is important about working on the feet?

8

Sports Massage for Side-Lying Positions

Most people who receive massages are asked to lie in prone and supine positions; few experience the side-lying position. As a sports and remedial massage therapist, you will be required to access muscles using a variety of approaches and techniques, making the side-lying position common and essential. I recommend getting used to working in this position by working entire massage sessions with clients in the side-lying position.

When clients are in the side-lying (laterally recumbent) position, you will need extra towels to manage their privacy as well as cushions or bolsters for support. Place bolsters or cushions under the client's head and the knee of the top leg. Position your client's bottom leg straight, in line with his torso, and the top leg at a 90-degree angle. You can also ask your client to hold the edge of the couch for further stability.

TIP Because the side-lying position does have a tendency to close up the area between the ribs and hip, you can place another cushion or a rolled-up towel just above the iliac crest to open up the area and make it easier to work between the ribs. This will also help you to gain access to the quadratus lumborum, which is an important side-bending muscle and slight torso rotator.

CLIENT TALK

Side-lying is used for a number of reasons, one of which includes the ability to access muscles that are located deep beneath the more superficial muscles. For example, if I want to access the muscles behind the gastrocnemius it is much easier as this position allows the tissue to drop away from the skeletal structure. I also use it for encouraging the muscles to separate from one another by working with gravity, allowing the tissue to drop away, and using techniques like transverse effleurage to help separate the adhered tissue.

On the following pages are instructions for a variety of sports massage techniques that can be used while your client is in the side-lying position.

Neck Massage Technique 1

Sit on the massage couch behind your client just below her shoulders. You should be far enough away to maintain an upright sitting position but close enough to be able to hold her shoulder with one hand while moving the other arm away from you along the lateral border of the neck all the way to the base of the skull without overreaching. You can work with a pillow under the client's head or without one. Removing the pillow will expose the working area more, but you should make sure your client is not in any discomfort. Be mindful of the sensitive nature of the neck as you choose how much depth and pressure to apply. Keep checking with your client verbally and observe her reactions.

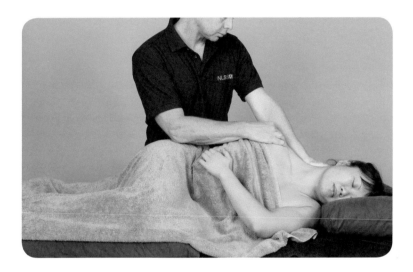

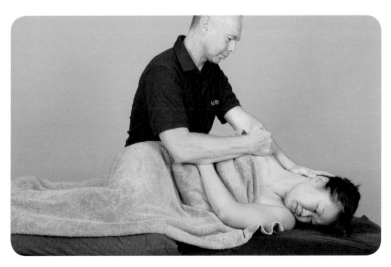

TIP If your hand slips on the shoulder because the lotion has made it slippery, use a towel to hold the shoulder while applying the stroke.

Neck Massage Technique 2

Standing behind your client's head with one arm stretched out, press the client's shoulder with this hand. With the other hand apply transverse or longitudinal strokes on the upper trapezius area. Keep a continuous alignment of your own legs and torso when applying these strokes.

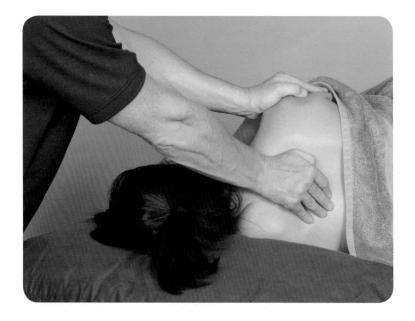

Shoulder and Arm Massage Technique 1

Standing behind and near the top of the client's head and using a bent arm, place your client's arm in yours, tucking it into your side to secure it. If the couch height is correct and your shoulders are relaxed, this position should be effortless. From here you can apply long strokes down the arm, working towards the chest or the length of the lateral side of the body.

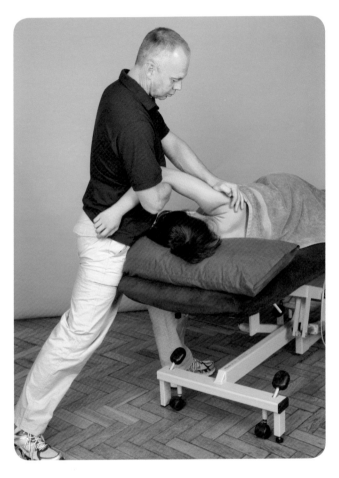

TIP To ensure an even and secure stroke while moving along the side of the client's body, use your legs to create the force of the movement while slightly pulling the arm tucked in at your side in the opposite direction.

Shoulder and Arm Massage Technique 2

To massage around the scapula and access the edges of the subscapularis underneath, start off by taking a wide stance with your legs behind your client's upper body. Place one hand on the anterior portion of the shoulder and massage the medial border of the scapula with the digits of the other hand. You can also use the first hand to push the shoulder back and down while using the pressure of the other hand to press up and under the scapula.

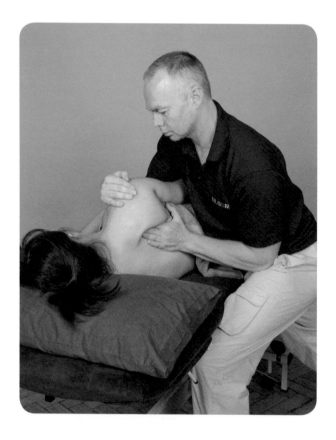

Torso Massage Technique 1

Stand behind your client facing towards her upper torso. Using a wide asymmetrical stance, put the hand closer to the midline of the client's body on her hip to stabilise her. Now take the outside hand and apply a long stroke up the erector spinae avoiding the spinous processes. Use your legs to generate the momentum of the movement, allowing your front knee to bend as you move forward. Maintain a flat back in alignment with your legs and head.

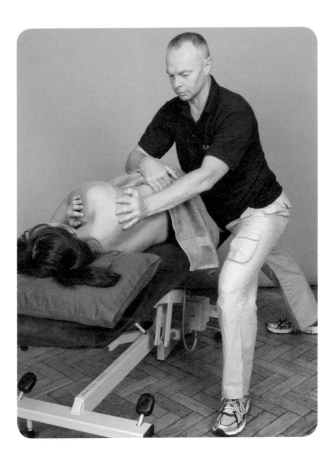

Torso Massage Technique 2

You can apply petrissage while standing on the other side of the client by gathering the tissue in a circular fashion, picking up and lifting the tissue. The key is to either use the couch as a prop to stabilise yourself (push your thighs into it) or engage your own abdominal muscles to create the force.

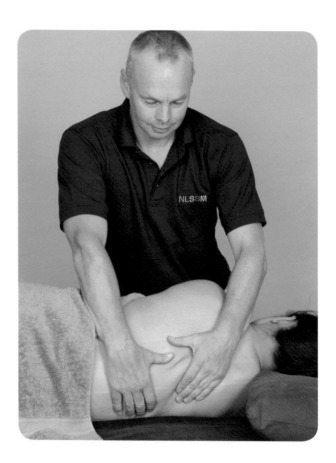

When working on the pelvis in the side-lying position, remember to lower the couch. The difference between the height of the client's pelvis in prone and side-lying positions is significant.

Pelvis Massage Technique 1

Stabilise the client's hip with one hand while using the other to apply the stroke, directing movement and strength from your legs. Relax your shoulders and extend your arm, using circular, transverse or longitudinal strokes. Your forearm and elbow can also be powerful tools in this position because they allow you to apply deeper strokes without compromising your working posture. If you choose to use either of these variations, maintain your postural alignment and be aware of the increased depth that can be generated with these choices. Watch out for client discomfort and work slower.

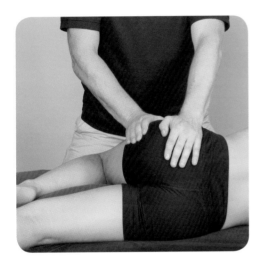
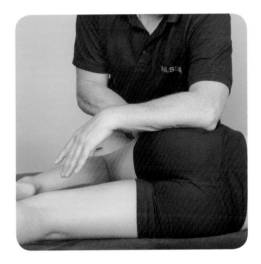
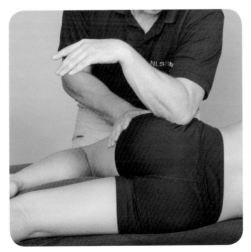

TIP If you choose to use either your elbow or your forearm, keep your hand and wrist relaxed by letting the hand hang loosely. This will keep the movement less invasive and rigid.

Thigh Massage Technique 1

This technique is appropriate for the outer thigh. When applying strokes along the outer thigh, control the depth of pressure because this can be quite painful. By angling your wrist at approximately 45 degrees rather than at 90 degrees, you will be less likely to compress the tissue into the bone; rather, you will comfortably push the tissue up the length of the thigh. Standing away from the movement by using an extended arm, use your legs to push the tissue along the thigh. You can approach this portion of the leg from two directions and apply a longitudinal or transverse stroke.

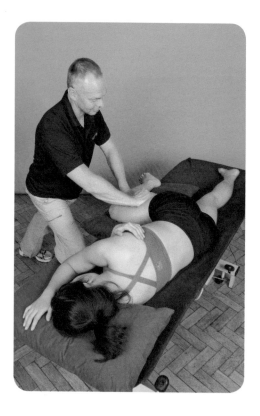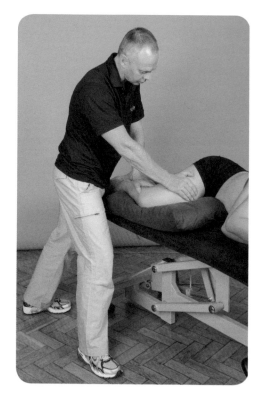

Thigh Massage Technique 2

This technique is appropriate for both the thigh and the leg. Place the leg that the client is resting on straight and move the top leg to a 90-degree angle. This creates a stable position in which to work. Put a pillow under the full length of the bent leg to help support it and even up the angle of the hips so the client's torso is straight. In this position you have access to both the top and bottom leg and can apply a variety of techniques transversely or longitudinally.

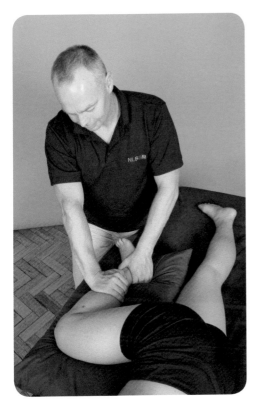 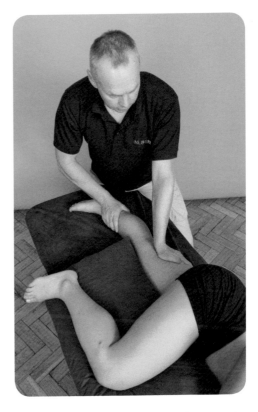

TIP Remember to change the position of your legs when you change from working on the lower portion of the leg to working on the upper thigh. Readjust your working position appropriately (i.e., to work on the upper thigh you will need to face the table; to work on the lower leg you will need to face towards the head of the couch). In both positions, assume an asymmetrical stance.

Quick Questions

1. Where would you place pillows or cushions for a client in a side-lying position?
2. Why do you have to lower the height of the couch when a client is in a side-lying position?
3. When is it appropriate to use the side-lying position?
4. Why should you place the client's top leg at 90 degrees and the bottom leg straight in a side-lying position?
5. What else can you suggest to the client to help stabilise her position?

PART IV

Sports Massage Programmes and Management

Chapter 9 is about developing your detective skills using consultation and physical assessment methods such as palpation, visual and movement tests. This will enable you to make suitable conclusions that will assist you in making the appropriate treatment goals. It is a process that needs to be revisited each time you see your client, hence it is useful to refer back to this chapter time and time again. Every session should contain elements of each of the assessment methods discussed in the chapter, but may not necessarily include them all.

Event work is an area in which sports massage therapists can gain valuable experience. Chapter 10 describes the different types of event massage and details what types of techniques are suitable, how long the massage should be, when it should take place and what considerations a therapist needs to look out for. If you are adventurous and are a good organizer you might be interested in the section "Organising an Event."

Chapter 11 delivers a general overview of the various classifications and common conditions that are included in disability sport, such as the Paralympic Games. The chapter provides an introduction about the physiological and physical demands that are placed on the athlete. It also addresses therapy considerations and modifications that are necessary in order to provide an appropriate treatment to meet athletes' needs.

9

Client Assessment

Client assessment can be divided into subjective, objective and interpretive stages. During the subjective assessment stage, you obtain information through written and verbal communication. This is considered the history-taking stage. Objective assessment includes tests and visual observation. This stage is the hands-on part of the evaluation that includes palpation and assessing range of motion. During the interpretive assessment stage, you compile and synthesize the information you have obtained, establish goals and plan the treatment. Evaluating and setting goals should be a part of every session because you will most likely have to modify your approach to treatment as you go along. It is important that you reevaluate the situation from session to session and even within a session to ensure that you are responding appropriately to your client's needs.

Subjective Assessment

During the subjective assessment, you need to identify any contraindications for treatment and gather relevant data about the client's training, lifestyle and goals. You must also determine areas that need to be worked on while establishing a baseline from which to measure the effectiveness of the treatment. Because the way you gather information will affect the quantity and quality of that information, you need good communication and detective skills.

Communication

Taking a thorough case history requires good communication and listening skills. To be an effective detective, you need a variety of verbal and non-verbal skills. The first step in being a good communicator is giving your full attention to the client and being able to focus on her needs. If you find you are finishing your client's sentences or are talking before she has finished speaking, you need to slow down your mind. Wait until she has finished explaining herself, and then clarify your understanding by summarising what you think she has said.

Also essential in gathering information from your clients are non-verbal cues such as facial expressions and how they hold their bodies. These can give you important clues about what they are not saying and how they are feeling. Gestures can also indicate the condition of the soft tissue; for example, if a client uses a pulling action with the hands, this might indicate that the tissue feels tight and needs to be stretched.

Client History

A client's medical history includes information about his past injuries, illnesses and surgeries (see figure 9.1 on page 116 for a medical history form). This can give valuable information and can often indicate what has influenced the current state of health of the soft tissue. The best method of getting this information is an interview. Giving a form to a client to fill in prior to the session can save time, but it removes the opportunity for good detective work. The questions in figure 9.2 on page 117 can help you prepare for this interview.

A client interview gives you the time to develop a therapeutic relationship and observe non-verbal cues. During the interview you should also find out the following:

- Personal identification and contact details. Try to get all of the client's phone numbers and an e-mail address in case you need to contact her quickly.

- Current health information, both physically and psychologically. Being particularly stressed by family life or a job can influence a client's current physical health.

- Current state of soft tissue health (acute, chronic or acute/chronic). If a client has a chronic condition that has become acute, you would manage the acute stage first and then address the chronic condition.

- The client's training regime or level of activity: how often, what type, how much time she spends training and the intensity. Also find out about her rest days, if she takes any.

- How the client spends a majority of her time. Consider the impact her activity is having on her muscle development and how it is influencing her posture and movement.

- Any other intrinsic and extrinsic factors that might have an effect on the client's condition (e.g., age, gender, equipment).

- What the client hopes to get from the session, where she wants to be and her short-term and long-term goals.

MEDICAL HISTORY

Name:	Tel. no. (home):	Tel. no. (work):
Address:	Mobile no.:	Date of birth:

Dr's name/tel. no.:

Address:

Occupation:	Weight:	Height:
Current medication(s):	Referred?	
Recent operations or illnesses:	Pregnancy:	

Circulation problems: (heart, pulmonary oedema, high/low blood pressure, poor circulation)	
Respiratory system: (asthma, bronchitis, hay fever)	
Skin disorders: (dermatitis, eczema, sensitivity, fungal infections)	
Muscular or skeletal problems: (fibromyalgia, previous fractures)	
Neurological problems: (sciatica, epilepsy, migraine)	
Urinary problems: (cystitis, thrush, kidney problems)	
Immune system: (prone to colds, reduced immune status)	
Gynaecological problems: (PMT, menopause, HRT, irregular periods)	
Hormonal problems: (diabetes)	
Digestive problems: (indigestion, constipation, IBS)	
Stress-related or psychological problems: (depression, anxiety, panic attacks, mood swings)	

INDEMNITY: I confirm to the best of my knowledge that I have not withheld any information relevant to my treatment and that I understand and accept full responsibility for the treatment that I am given. I also agree that I have given the correct information as detailed on this form, and should inform the therapist should these circumstances change.

Client signature:_____

Therapist signature:_____ Date:_____

Figure 9.1 Every client should complete a medical history form.

From S. Findlay, 2010, *Sports massage* (Champaign, IL: Human Kinetics). Reprinted, by permission, from J. Johnson, 2009, *Soft tissue release* (Champaign, IL: Human Kinetics), 139.

INITIAL QUESTIONS

Client Name:	Date:

1. **How may I help?**

2. **Where is the discomfort you described?**

3. **When did it start?**

4. **How was it caused?**

5. **Is it getting better, worse or staying the same?**

6. **Does anything make it worse?**

7. **Does anything make it better?**

8. **Have you had previous treatment for this complaint? Was it helpful?**

9. **Have you had this condition before?**

10. **Have you had any previous injuries to the same area?**

11. **Can you describe the type of discomfort you are feeling?**

12. **How does this condition affect your work and leisure?**

13. **Is there anything else you think I need to know?**

Figure 9.2 Use these initial questions to identify the reason for treatment and to assess the client's medical history.

From S. Findlay, 2010, *Sports massage* (Champaign, IL: Human Kinetics). Reprinted, by permission, from J. Johnson, 2009, *Soft tissue release* (Champaign, IL: Human Kinetics), 133.

To design an appropriate treatment plan, you will need to consider any intrinsic and extrinsic factors that might have had an influence in the development of the client's condition. Intrinsic factors typically are related to the internal make-up of a person, whereas extrinsic factors are external situations that can influence the development of injury. The following are examples of various conditions for both:

Intrinsic

- Physical fitness—What is their state of health?
- Body composition—Are they suited for their chosen sport?
- Training technique—Do they have the support of a good coach, or are they training ad hoc?
- Anatomic variants—Do they have leg length differences, or are they bow legged?
- Age—Does their age dictate certain nutritional requirement or healing rates?
- Gender—Are there anatomical and physiological influences?
- Past injuries—How have past injuries been resolved, if at all, and how have they influenced current muscle function?
- Psychological predisposition—Do they have good or bad memories? What is their personality type?

Extrinsic

- Equipment—Are they wearing any, and is it in good order?
- Environment—What are the weather, altitude, and surface conditions?
- Training FITT (frequency, intensity, time and type)—Have they trained adequately and appropriately for this event?
- Competition—Is it the beginning of the season, and are they nervous or pumped up?

Subjective Questions

Clients do not always divulge all the necessary information in their case histories. For personal reasons they might not feel comfortable telling all, they may not believe certain information is important or relevant, or they may simply have forgotten about it. To get all the information you need, continue to ask questions during massage sessions, especially if you sense that the information the client has given does not correspond to your findings. The following questions can help you investigate a chronic condition, one that might have acute elements involved. If the condition presents as an acute injury, the questions should be more focused on the nature and symptoms of inflammation and pain.

- Where is the injury? Can you show me?
- When did it occur? If unknown: When do you think it first started?

- What are the details about the onset of injury? Was it sudden, traumatic, or slow in developing?
- What are the signs and symptoms now?

- Can you describe your main problems and activities of daily living?

- How is this affecting your sport?

- What aggravates your symptoms?

- What eases your symptoms?

- Do you have any discomfort? Can you describe it for me?

- Are you taking any medications for it?

- Are there any previous conditions that might have influenced this one?

- Have you had this injury before?

- Is the condition improving or getting worse?

- Have you had any treatment for this condition? If so, what did you have and was it effective?

- What investigations did you have and what were the results?

- What does your training regime consist of?

- What do you hope to accomplish by seeking sports massage?

- What specific goals do you have, both short term and long term?

CLIENT TALK

Once, while massaging a client's lower leg, the tension and muscle development that I felt could not be fully explained by the sport and position she played. When I asked her about this, she remarked that she had worn braces as a child. She did not understand the importance of this and how it was influencing her muscle development and behaviour to this day. Lesson learnt: keep asking questions.

Objective Assessment

Once you have gathered all the verbal and written information, you can move on to the functional component of the case history. Assessments that are typically included are palpation of the soft tissue, pain assessment, postural assessment, range of motion testing and muscle function testing. (Functional gait analysis and a biomechanical assessment are important components of an assessment process, but require a more advanced training background and practical experience and are beyond the scope of this book.)

Using a variety of assessment tools will help you to 'prove it or lose it' in your final analysis. Each bit of information on its own does not mean much, so it is important to make your decisions based on a global evaluation rather than an isolated one. In medicine, one of the principles of investigation used to determine the patient's condition is through a process of elimination. This is done by sending a patient for a series of tests to either prove or disprove their state of health. In sports massage, we are doing a similar thing by using a variety of tests to try to prove or disprove the possible reasons for the presenting symptoms. The order in which you do these assessments is up to you. Keep in mind that clients generally do not want to have to move about a great deal; many have the preconceived idea that massage consists of prone and supine positions. Working in a logical manner helps to minimise the number of times you have to reposition your client, thereby helping maintain a relaxed state of mind and body.

Palpation

Palpation is the primary tool of a massage therapist. The feedback gained from touching the soft tissue is essential in making an informed decision about what the problems are and how you are going to treat them. The skill in palpation comes from slow and thoughtful movements, starting off superficially and moving into deeper tissue and working from a general approach to a more specific one. This reveals more information, allowing for a more considered plan of action.

Client feedback is vital, especially if there is an area of tenderness. During the examination process it is important to contrast bilaterally. Start by assessing the unaffected side to give you an idea of what is normal. Initially, you are looking for superficial changes, including the following:

- Skin changes (i.e., bruises, rough-ness, colour)
- Temperature changes (hot [inflammation] or cold [ischemia])
- Superficial muscle hypertonicity
- Fascial restrictions, decreased movement
- Adhesions (tissue feels stuck together)

- Tenderness
- Oedema or swelling
- Hills and valleys (muscle or structural differences)
- Skin drag (i.e., sticky)
- Hydration (dry or damp)

TIP During your visual assessment, make note of any moles and keep a record of them so you can assess for any changes in their size, shape, colour and texture. This is especially useful for moles on the back because people don't usually inspect this area.

Following your superficial observations, progress your palpation to the deeper structures to assess the following:

- Soft tissue mobility
- Tenderness
- Oedema (congested or boggy/chronic, hard/acute)

- Deep muscle or fascial tension
- Fibrosis (scars)
- Trigger points

Allow yourself to become quiet during the palpation process. Close your eyes and let your fingers take over. This will increase your sensitivity and your findings.

Pain Assessment

Pain is a very individual experience. Because each person's understanding of, tolerance of and coping mechanisms for pain are unique, pain assessment can be challenging. For this reason, you must remain sensitive to the individual client's needs and work within his capacity. When you apply pressure to the tissue and the client tells you that it feels good, this indicates that the pressure is producing an analgesic effect and the client usually wants you to continue in this way. Harmful pain is indicated by a muscle contraction or the client pushing against the movement you are applying. The more vocal client will verbalise her feelings and tell you when it hurts (it is inappropriate to tell a client that this type of pain is good for her). Other indicators that your client is experiencing discomfort ranges from sweating, shallow breathing or holding her breath, clenching her fists or fidgeting in other body parts. As mentioned before, verbal cues are an obvious clue, but clients can also become very quiet, and a few react with laughter. During the assessment process, ensure that there are no factors that would suppress a client's ability to feel pain, such as medication or diseases such as diabetes.

When assessing pain, try to determine as accurately as possible which structure is affected. Table 9.1 will help you to isolate the structure that might be involved by comparing the various types of soft tissue response to pain; when a client might feel it; whether it is at the start of the movement or the end; and whether the client feels it during an active, resisted or passive movement.

The body naturally reacts to avoid pain by minimising movement or stress to the area. This occurs by stabilising the injured area and applying 'muscle guarding', or splinting, whereby the body places itself into a position of ease, an unnatural body position. This creates a compensatory pattern throughout the body to accommodate the changes in muscle usage. If this change is not dealt with or corrected, it can become an established pattern leading to secondary problems. One of the jobs of a massage therapist can be unravelling these compensatory patterns. The key to reestablishing and encouraging new patterns is to work methodically and slowly; otherwise, the tissue can react by reengaging the muscle guarding response.

Table 9.1   Pain Behaviour of Damaged Tissue

	Active	Active resisted	Passive
Muscle	Pain on initiation of the movement involving the contraction of that muscle	Pain on initiation of the movement involving the contraction of that muscle	Pain on the passive stretch of that muscle
Tendon	Pain on initiation of the movement involving the contraction of that muscle	Pain on initiation of the movement involving the contraction of that muscle	Pain on the passive stretch of that muscle differentiated from muscle problems by the location of the pain
Ligament	Pain at the end of the range when the ligament is stretched	No pain	Pain at the end of the range when the ligament is stretched
Joint capsule	Pain at the end of many ranges (and the range may be reduced by adhesions)	No pain unless the capsule is swollen; then there is pain when the muscle is contracted as a result of compression or tension	Pain at the end of many ranges (and the range may be reduced by adhesions)

Factors that can influence a person's ability to tolerate pain include personality, socio-cultural background, previous experience and current state of health. Understanding how these factors can affect your client's feelings and reaction to pain will guide you to select and perform techniques with greater accuracy.

TIP A valuable tool to help determine whether the tissue is healthy enough to receive mas-sage is to apply slow pressure to the area with your thumb. If the pain subsides within 10 seconds, massage is fine; if the pain increases during the 10 seconds, the situation is too acute and you should implement protocols for an acute stage.

The following principles will help you return the soft tissue to a healthy condition. First, allow the tissues to dictate the speed at which you move; wait until it relaxes and gives way to your touch before moving on. If you move too quickly, you can create unnecessary pain and also damage the tissue. Do not over treat an area; always keep in mind that less is more. Follow all your work with flushing and relaxation techniques to assist with the healing process. Always respect what your client tells you about how he feels about pain, and remain empathetic. Clients are the best source of information and can direct you about when to lighten up or slow down. By applying these principles, you will have a more positive outcome.

TIP Keep the following in mind when massaging:

- Less is more
- Do not over treat
- Flush the area
- Work in cooperation with the tissue
- Respect the client's feedback
- Slow down, feel the response
- Light can be deep

PAIN SCALE   Pain tolerance is different from a pain threshold. A pain threshold is the starting point at which a person begins to feel pain, and pain tolerance is more about how much pain a person can cope with. A pain scale is a useful way to measure this pain threshold. It allows you to gauge the levels of pain before, during and after each treatment as well as from session to session. It is a practical way of measuring and reinforcing progression; when the healing process seems slow, the client can see that there is a change and remain hopeful. (Of course, this only works if there is actually a positive change.) You can use pain scales in a variety of ways. One way is to get verbal feedback from the client indicating mild, moderate or severe pain. Another is moni-toring the measurement of pain using a scale of 0 to 10, with 0 being no pain and 10 being intolerable pain.

It is useful to monitor the pain or discomfort levels throughout your treatment to get a clear idea of the intensity at which you are working (ideally, nothing above an 8, preferably around a 6 or 7). Your client can best indicate what is comfortable for him and guide you to the depth and speed of work that best suits him.

SUBJECTIVE QUESTIONS   This section is addressing pain specifically, but what a client feels might not be pain per se. Initially, it is more prudent to ask a client what she is experiencing—that is, how the symptoms manifest. Allow her to name it or describe it in her own words. This gives you an honest account of what she is feeling. The following questions are specific to the assessment of pain, but other words such as *discomfort* can also be used if this is what your client is experiencing.

- How and when did your pain (discomfort) start? Did it come on slowly or suddenly?
- What does it feel like? Can you describe it?
- What is the severity on a scale of 1 to 10?
- What makes it worse?
- What makes it better? Are there relieving factors such as the following:

  Movement (chronic tension)

  Rest (acute)

  Position (indicator of cause)

  Hot (muscular)

  Cold (inflammation)
- Does it vary during the day? If so, when?
- What is the frequency—every day, all the time, intermittent?
- Has it gotten better or worse over time, or is it much the same?
- What do you think is causing it?
- Does it radiate anywhere?
- Are there any associated factors?
- What tests or investigations have you had for the pain (e.g., X-rays, scans, blood tests, nerve tests)?
- What treatment, if any, are you having or have you had in the past? Has it been effective?
- How has this pain (discomfort) affected your training?
- Do you suffer from any other medical condition not related to it, or are you receiving medical treatment, including medicines, from your doctor?
- Are you waiting to see any other specialists or to have an operation because of it?

DESCRIPTORS   Pain descriptors can be a valuable tool to help evaluate and establish a clear picture of a condition. Pain as a diagnostic tool on its own is inadequate and by no means will give you all the information you need, but it is important that you do a thorough evaluation so you can make informed decisions. In some circumstances it is more appropriate to refer the client to another health care provider based on the description of the condition. The following descriptors will give you some direction about which systems might be affected or the condition the pain might be associated with.

Sharp—Acute, might also be associated with a neural condition.

Dull—Bony, chronic condition.

Deep—Depending on the structure, it could be associated with a chronic, bony or neural condition.

Boring—Bony condition, arthritis or cancer.

Aching—Chronic condition.

Crawling—Autonomic or CNS-generated condition.

Burning—Fascial condition; can also indicate spinal cord damage, neural pain or fibromyalgia.

Diffuse—Possibility of non-muscular or referred muscular condition.

Throbbing—Vascular condition as well as acute inflammation.

Stinging—Dermal condition.

Lancing/linear/electric—Neural condition.

Colicky—Visceral condition.

RED FLAGS   Red flags are indicators that emergency medical treatment or urgent referral is needed. If your client demonstrates the following symptoms and they are associated with low back pain or sciatica, or the client has been in a recent car accident, it is advisable to refer her on. A certain degree of clinical judgment is required because these symptoms on their own would generally not pose a serious enough risk to warrant further referral. If in doubt, it is better to err on the side of caution and refer.

Headaches—Especially concerning if there are no obvious musculoskeletal factors.

Numbness—Neural or vascular issues.

Pins and needles—Neural or vascular issues.

Palpitations—Cardiovascular condition.

Dizziness.

Disturbed sleep.

Symptoms with coughing and sneezing —Spinal condition.

Bearing down—Spinal condition.

Changes in bowel or urinary function—Cauda equina or a possible neurological condition.

Postural Assessment

A person with ideal posture moves in an effortless manner, has no pain and is able to meet reasonable physical demands. He can make efficient use of the musculoskeletal system wherein there exists a state of balance between how the muscles work and joint loading.

There is a lot of discussion about the functions and roles of postural muscles, phasic muscles, and how these types of muscles behave when they become dysfunctional. Postural muscles often function at a low level of tension over long periods without tiring. Current belief is that when these muscles develop imbalances, they tend to shorten and become hyperactive. Phasic muscles, which are the mobilisers, tend to weaken, become inactive and sometimes lengthen (see Chaitow & Delany *Clinical Applications of Neuromuscular Techniques* Vol 1 (2nd Edition) p. 36). In both situations, the normal function of the muscle is altered affecting its alignment and disrupting the equilibrium of the joints, thus resulting in a faulty posture.

A significant increase in joint load can cause muscular imbalances. These imbalances can lead to health and soft tissue problems that can interfere with an athlete's performance. The following factors can lead to muscle imbalances and poor posture:

- Faulty biomechanics
- Previous injury
- Psychosocial issues
- Demands of the sport or everyday activities
- Combination of the preceding

Conditions that might arise from the misuse, abuse or disuse of the musculoskeletal system are fascial restrictions, compensation patterns, under- or overdevelopment of the soft tissue and the misalignment of some structures. These conditions will reflect in the length and balance patterns of the muscle and will need to be considered when making any treatment decisions.

To make choices about which muscles to target and what techniques to use, you must understand muscle behaviour. A general rule is to loosen a tight muscle before strengthening surrounding ones; any changes in tension of the target muscle will affect the behaviour of its neighbours. Therefore, if you choose to alter the condition of the soft tissue, you will need to consider the effect it will have elsewhere. It is important to execute a carefully considered and thoughtful plan, work gradually, allow the body time to make adaptations without causing unfavourable instability and assess and reassess for changes. This will help to ensure that the changes you elicit are the intended ones.

ASSESSMENT   A postural assessment starts the moment your client walks through the door. This is a prime opportunity to observe her natural movement, how she holds herself, her facial expressions and her general energy levels. This unofficial observation period allows you to witness your client's everyday behaviour. Clients tend to change their behaviour (such as pulling themselves more upright) once they know they are being observed.

At the start of your training a plumb line can help you see musculoskeletal changes. This tool is useful until you have developed a natural eye that can pick up any differences or unusual changes through casual observation.

TIP As soon as a client believes she is being observed, she tends to place herself in a position that she believes is correct, rather than in a natural manner. Bear in mind your client's feelings and her reaction to having a pair of eyes scrutinise her; she might be finding the whole process a bit intimidating. To encourage a more relaxed state, try not to directly stare at your client's posture, but casually look while keeping up comfortable conversation. Keep your assessment time to a minimum.

To do a postural assessment using a plumb line, ask your client to stand and then place a plumb line the length of his body. This allows you to assess the bony and soft tissue landmarks in relation to vertical and horizontal reference lines. A plumb line is not hard to put together: take a length of string, place a weight at the end and hang it somewhere that will allow for a lateral, anterior and posterior view of the client. Posterior, anterior and lateral postural assessments are outlined on pages 126-128.

TIP If your client assumes a wide stance or stands in a forced unnatural position, ask her to march on the spot about 10 times. This will usually bring her back to a more natural position.

POSTERIOR VIEW

Ask the client to stand with feet apart in a natural position. Make sure the plumb line falls midway between the heels and that the client's body does not touch the line.

Observations

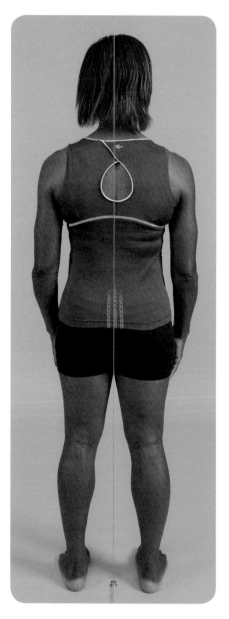

Yes	No	Are the shoulders level?
Yes	No	Are the height and positions of the scapulae equal? Is there any 'winging'?
Yes	No	Is there a lateral curvature of the spine?
Yes	No	Is the head tilted to one side? Right or left?
Yes	No	Are both arm positions symmetrical?
Yes	No	Are the fat folds (creases) at the sides equal in number and symmetrical?
Yes	No	Are the pelvic crests level?
Yes	No	Are the paravertebral muscles built up?
Yes	No	Are the buttock creases level?
Yes	No	Are the creases of the knees equal in height?
Yes	No	Are the feet placed symmetrically apart?
Yes	No	Do the Achilles tendons appear deviated or symmetrical?
Yes	No	Are the positions of the malleoli symmetrical in relation to the heels?

From S. Findlay, 2010, *Sports massage* (Champaign, IL: Human Kinetics).

ANTERIOR VIEW

Ask the client to stand with feet apart in a natural position. Make sure the plumb line falls midway between the heels and that the client's body does not touch the line.

Observations

Yes　No　Is the head tilted to one side? Right or left?

Yes　No　Are the shoulder levels symmetrical?

Yes　No　Is the clavicular line horizontal?

Yes　No　Are fingertips at an equal point at the side of the body?

Yes　No　Are the pelvic crests level?

Yes　No　Are the patellae deviated? Laterally or medially?

Yes　No　Do the feet have a normal arch? Are they flat or high arched?

Yes　No　Do the feet pronate?

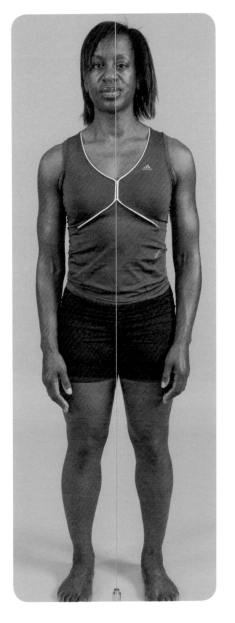

From S. Findlay, 2010, *Sports massage* (Champaign, IL: Human Kinetics).

LATERAL VIEW

Position your client so the plumb line is passing just in front of the lateral malleolus. Ideally, the line should then run as follows:

- Slightly anterior to the ankle
- Slightly anterior to the centre of the knee
- Just posterior to the centre of the hip joint
- Through the centre of the shoulder joint
- Through the ear lobe

Observations

Yes	No	Is the head balanced?
Yes	No	Are the shoulders protracted?
Yes	No	Are the normal spinal curves exaggerated? Is the client lordotic or kyphotic?
Yes	No	Are the normal spinal curves reversed?
Yes	No	Are the arm positions at the sides of the body? Behind or in front?
Yes	No	Are the knees relaxed?
Yes	No	Are the knees locked in extension?
Yes	No	Is the body rotated as a whole?

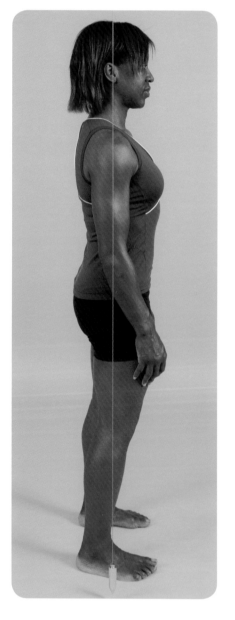

From S. Findlay, 2010, *Sports massage* (Champaign, IL: Human Kinetics).

Slight deviations from side to side are normal. No body is symmetrical, and it is not unusual when comparing one side to another to find some discrepancies. What you are looking for are normal shapes, placement and similarities.

The information gathered from a postural assessment will give you a greater understanding about where the stresses are being placed on the musculoskeletal system. What you do with your findings will depend on what the problem is and the intended goals of treatment. Your final analysis will need to include all of your other assessments so you can create an accurate treatment plan.

Range of Motion Testing and Muscle Function

The purpose of range of motion (ROM) testing is to help you make informed decisions about which muscles to target to create a beneficial balance. Sometimes it is inappropriate to lengthen or lessen the tension in a structure because its purpose is to stabilise a joint or help in the performance of the athlete. Therefore, you must understand which muscles hinder and which enhance an athlete's performance. Involvement with athletes requires a thorough understanding of movement, which is beyond the scope of this book. This section provides a basic understanding and is intended to assist you in developing an awareness of the assessment skills needed to test for normal and abnormal ROM, muscle function and strength. It will help you determine restrictions and weaknesses, as well as assist you in measuring improvements.

TIP ROM tests assess the following:

- Increased or decreased ROM
- Pain
- Increased or decreased strength
- Ease of movement
- End of joint feel
- Bind
- Crepitus

When assessing the muscular system, keep in mind that it acts as one complete, interactive unit rather than as independent muscles. Any imbalance in one area of the musculoskeletal system affects other structures elsewhere in the body. This is why it is always important when assessing a client to take a global overview of soft tissue function rather than focus on an individual muscle or joint. No one muscle is designed to absorb all the stress of the body; muscle behaviour is meant to be a combined balance of function. As sport necessitates repetitive actions and can constitute asymmetrical movements, these actions can often disrupt normal balance and place greater demands on some structures that can lead to an increased risk of injury.

Stress can also result from previous injury, microtrauma, postural changes and emotional stress. In the case of microtrauma, injury can go unnoticed. Within a small area adhesions can form, placing stress on the surrounding tissue. Although at first these adhesions are microscopic, they can interfere with the normal function of the tissue and cause further tissue breakdown in the surrounding areas. Eventually, this can develop into a more substantial issue.

Consider the example of a runner who complains of knee pain and lower back discomfort. Originally, the symptoms were almost non-existent; it all started off as a bit of a twinge in both calves 6 months ago. The twinge did not happen all the time, but every so often after running he felt his calves were tight. Eventually, the discomfort progressed to being a regular feature after every run and increased to include an uncomfortable tension when he started out but would disappear shortly after his muscles warmed up. After a few months he was not able to bear weight or put his heel down first thing in the morning. It was taking longer and longer for the discomfort to ease off when first beginning a run. He recently noticed that he was avoiding putting his heel down when running and was now unable to run without knee pain. His symptoms have now progressed to include lower back problems.

This illustrates how microtrauma can evolve from a bit of tension to a more global problem. The preceding scenario demonstrates that as muscle function and tissue deteriorate, compensatory patterns develop. Massage can play a vital role in preventing such conditions by breaking down adhesions and lessening muscle tension using soft tissue techniques.

ACTIVE AND PASSIVE ROM TESTING   The purpose of ROM testing is to determine a client's range of motion both actively and passively. You are assessing for the feel (e.g., whether it moves easily or is stiff) as well as the distance a person can move. The assessment should identify any pain, limited movement or unusual grating sounds (crepitus).

In an active test the client makes the movement. This has the advantage of allowing you to estimate the client's comfort range. An active ROM test can also help distinguish between joint and muscular pain. Feeling pain in an active movement more than likely indicates a soft tissue issue (i.e., muscle or tendon). Feeling pain in a passive movement more than likely indicates skeletal pain associated with a joint or bone.

In both active and passive ROM testing, the client is taken through a normal range of motion. In active testing you record what the client is willing or able to do. Passive testing identifies limited and excessive ROM and allows you to assess for strength, ease of movement, how the joint feels during the movement, end feel and bind. If there is any pain during passive testing, you should stop the movement at that point.

Range of Motion   Each range of movement tested is measured from the neutral line of the anatomic position and taken through the sagittal, frontal and transverse planes. These tests should reflect the normal movement that is available for that joint (i.e., flexion, extension, rotation, abduction, adduction and circumduction). Any ROM that is greater than the expected degree is considered hypermobile; anything less represents a restriction and is considered hypomobile. Always compare limbs and joints on both sides of the body.

The ROM photos on pages 131-132 show a few basic tests to help you evaluate what is normal for a client and enable you to compare your findings. They illustrate the most common range of motion tests and address the differing opinions about what are considered accepted ranges. These photos lay the foundation for assessing clients, but you must keep in mind what might be the normal ROM for individual clients might not be the same for everyone.

Basic Range of Motion Tests

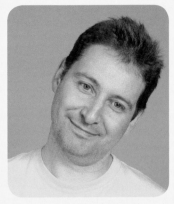

40-45 degrees of lateral neck flexion.

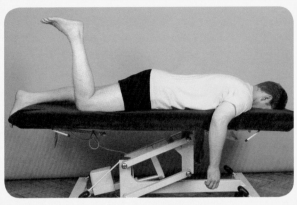

90-140 degrees of knee flexion.

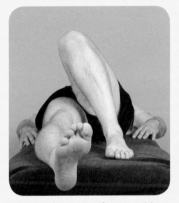

35-40 degrees of internal hip rotation.

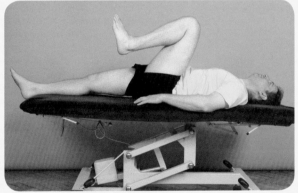

130-135 degrees of hip flexion.

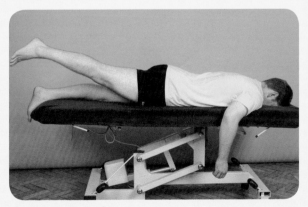

10-30 degrees of hip extension.

»continued

Basic Range of Motion Tests »continued

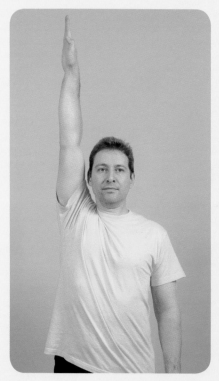
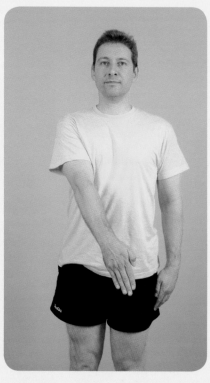

180 degrees of shoulder abduction.   50 degrees of shoulder adduction.

Normal and Abnormal Findings   A person's normal end of range is limited by muscles, tendons, structures within the joint such as ligaments, or the bones themselves. In a test for soft tissue stretch (as in a straight-leg hamstring stretch), the tissue should have an increase of tension that feels springy or has a sensation of stretching an elastic band as it gets closer to its end range. If you are performing a test on a capsule (as in a shoulder), it should feel like stretching a piece of leather. End feel for bone (as in elbow extension) is as you would expect: hard and sudden. In all of these tests there should be no pain.

End of Range Tests

STRAIGHT-LEG HAMSTRING STRETCH   Place your client in a supine position. Remove all cushions and bolsters to allow the pelvis and body to lie in a neutral position. In an active stretch, the client lifts one leg straight up towards the head while the other one remains extended on the couch. Watch that the leg on the couch does not start to bend at the knee. Also keep an eye on the leg that you are lifting to make sure it remains straight. At the same time, be aware of what the pelvis is doing: Make sure it does not alter its position during the lift. There should be no pain during this procedure. If there is, stop the movement and assist the client to return his leg to the table. In a passive test the same process happens but you, the therapist, control the movement. Make sure you support the leg behind the knee in order to prevent any undue stress on the joint. Watch out for the same unwanted movements; if and when that happens, the test should be stopped because that is the point at which the client range of movement is limited.

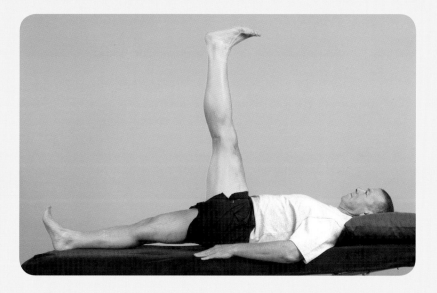

EXTERNAL AND INTERNAL SHOULDER ROTATION   Sit your client comfortably on the edge of the couch, making sure his feet are planted on the floor and his back is supported. This can be done by either placing a pillow between you and the client using your body to support him, or getting up on the couch on one bent leg while using the other bent leg to support the client from the side. In both an active and passive test, the client brings his arm up to shoulder height. Make sure he can do this without raising the shoulder; otherwise, only bring it up to the height that is comfortable for him. For both a medial or internal shoulder rotation test and a lateral or external test,

»continued

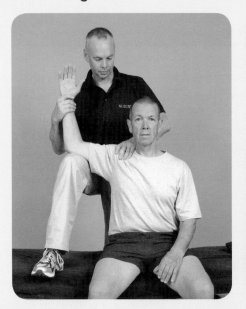
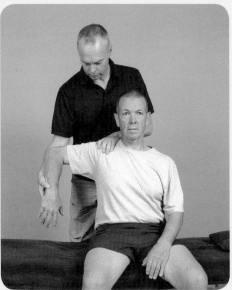

the client's arm is bent at the elbow to 90 degrees. Keeping this position, rotate the forearm either forward or backwards until a restriction is felt.

TIP If the client cannot raise his arm up so that the elbow is at the same height as the shoulder, he might have a shoulder impingement or Adhesive Capsulitus (Frozen Shoulder). Confirmation of either condition will need further investigation.

ELBOW EXTENSION This test, like the others, can be performed in a seated position or any other position that allows for full range of movement. In this particular test the arm is supported while the client is in a seated position on the couch. Take the arm out to the side assessing for abnormal sensations. A normal sensation would be a hard end feel as bone meets bone.

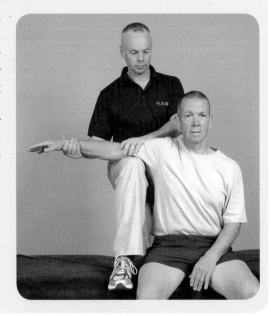

A restriction of the limb before its normal end range because of pain would indicate an abnormal finding. Regardless of whether it is due to a soft or hard tissue problem, you should stop any further movement at this point. Sometimes a muscle spasm occurs as a reflexive reaction to pain. End of range can be shortened as a result of fibrosis of the tissue without the presence of inflammation. As in the shoulder, the normal leathery end feel becomes tough and restricted. A soft or mushy feel indicates that oedema is present. You should refer the client to a health care specialist if there is no stabilisation within the joint, if you believe there is serious damage or if you feel an unusual springy or rebounding sensation within a joint.

Decreased range of movement can be caused by postural changes, fibrosis of the tissue, adhesions, muscle guarding, joint degeneration and other factors such as age and gender. Increased range can be a result of hypermobility or the instability of the joint as previously discussed.

If the restriction in motion is due to muscle guarding (to protect and stabilise the joint), be cautious. Make any changes gradually, allowing time for the tissues to adapt to the changes. Observing and evaluating the global effects of your soft tissue work is important to the success of your therapy.

TIP How to differentiate among acute, subacute and chronic conditions:

- Acute—Evidence of pain before the normal ROM is reached.
- Subacute—Pain is felt at the end of normal ROM.
- Chronic—Pain may be produced by applying a bit more pressure at the end of the active or passive ROM.

STRENGTH TESTING While assessing the range of motion of a limb, you can also test for strength as follows:

- First, stabilise any other body part that could become involved in the movement. This will help to isolate the muscle that you are targeting.
- Apply a small amount of resistance at the end of the lever system (e.g., to test the strength of knee flexion, place the hand on the client's heel while bringing it towards the hip).

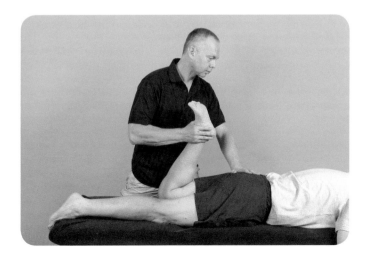

- Ask the client to move slowly as you apply a bit of resistance to control the movement. The muscles should be able to withstand the appropriate amount of resistance without pain for 10 to 30 seconds and without recruiting other muscles.
- Use palpation or visual assessment to make sure that the muscle you are targeting is the one that is engaged.
- Always compare both sides (e.g., both legs).

Contraindications for strength testing include acute pain, acute injury or trauma, inflammation and joint dysfunction.

A contraction that does not produce any pain and has an appropriate amount of strength indicates a normal strength finding. Pain during a strong contraction indicates an injury within the muscle, tendon or periosteal unit. A weak and painless contraction could indicate one of a number of dysfunctional conditions including poor gait, lack of use due to a hypertonic antagonist pattern, inhibition due to an injury to the adjacent joint structures, nerve irritation or impingement or a postural condition that has led to a length tension imbalance. Depending on your findings, apply massage in a considered manner to get the desired result.

Interpretive Stage

The interpretive assessment stage is about collating the information, identifying your client's needs and formulating a plan of action. The initial information you have gathered provides a base to work from, but you need to keep in mind that changes will happen from session to session and even during a single session. Therefore, you may need to return to the preceding tests at any time. Many factors will influence the direction your treatment will take, including client compliancy with recommendations, further information received and reaction to the massage. You must remain open and adaptable to any changes, positive or negative, and recognise when it is appropriate to reassess or reevaluate the situation.

Goal setting isn't so much about what massage techniques to use, but about determining the outcomes your client wants to achieve and how to get there. Goals should be specific and relevant to the person's sport or activity, and they need to be measurable and obtainable within a specified time period.

Following are examples of functional limitations and goals:

- *Functional limitation:* A runner is unable to run more than 5 miles because of pain in the Achilles tendon. *Goal:* The client will be able to run pain free for 5 miles.
- *Functional limitation:* A weightlifter is unable to dead lift more than 20 kilograms (44 lb) due to lower back pain. *Goal:* The client will be able to dead lift 20 kilograms (44 lb) of weight without complaints of pain.
- *Functional limitation:* A client is unable to brush her teeth because of pain that occurs when abducting her arm. *Goal:* The client will be able to brush her teeth pain free.

To design an appropriate treatment plan, you will need to consider all of the intrinsic and extrinsic factors that have influenced the development of the condition, as well as the information from your assessments and the client's case history. Avoid making any conclusive statements or goals; always leave room for other possibilities and considerations. Often, the presenting symptoms are not the whole story. Once you start to unravel the layers of soft tissue, you might find evidence that points you to a different conclusion. You must be able to respond and adapt.

Following are guidelines for establishing and implementing effective treatment goals:

- Set goals that are challenging yet realistic.
- Set goals that are specific, behavioural and measurable.
- Set both process and outcome goals.
- Use positive terminology.
- Establish a comprehensive timetable for goal completion.
- Monitor and evaluate progress.
- Focus on degrees of achievement.
- Make goals personal.

Goals can be divided into short-term, intermediate and long-term goals. By working with the client to combine both sport and life goals, you can help make the outcome more realistic and achievable.

Referral is an important consideration at the start of treatment or further into the treatment because clients may need further investigative tests as well as the help of other professionals in the fields of exercise, nutrition or psychology. Keep in mind the value of working with and learning from another professional; massage can be an isolating profession, and it is prudent to get further advice and recommendations.

It takes practice at all stages of assessment to become comfortable with the process and to develop the handling skills. Experience and practice will enable you to ask the right questions, move the client in a comfortable manner, know when to assess and what to assess, and accurately interpret the results and set appropriate goals. No textbook or teacher can teach you these skills. The best way to become proficient is to get out there and practise.

After you have set your overall goals, you can put together a plan of action. How you implement the plan will depend upon a number of factors such as what techniques you have in your tool box and which ones are suitable, as well as the time scale (i.e., do you have months, days or a single session). There also are the expectations of the client and a variety of intrinsic and extrinsic factors such as the client's health and age to consider. Throughout this process, keep in mind your aims as a sports massage therapist. Primarily, they are to keep an athlete injury free and to optimise muscle performance. As soft tissue therapists, we can have a very positive effect, but sometimes it is necessary and beneficial to work together, as a team, with other health care professionals or training staff. You should have a client-centred approach that allows the input of all available therapies to give your clients the best chance to achieve their goals.

TIP The client assessment form in figure 9.3 will help you synthesize all of the subjective, objective, and interpretive assessments you'll need to do to fully assess your clients.

Client name:		Date of birth:
Address:		Postal code:
Mobile:	Home:	Office:
E-mail:		
Occupation:		
Doctor's contact details:		Postal code:

Initial reason for coming:

Special considerations: (i.e., allergies, preferences)

Medical history:

Training schedule (FITT):

Frequency

Intensity

Time

Type

Initial interview summary:

Subjective findings

Objective findings

- Postural

- Range of motion

- Functional limitations

- Palpation

Interpretive findings

Figure 9.3 Client assessment form.

From S. Findlay, 2010, *Sports massage* (Champaign, IL: Human Kinetics).

Goals
Functional short-term goals:

Functional long-term goals:

Massage treatment plan:

Treatment:

Reassessment findings:

Pain or discomfort ratings:
Pre-massage   1 2 3 4 5 6 7 8 9 10

During massage   1 2 3 4 5 6 7 8 9 10

Post-massage   1 2 3 4 5 6 7 8 9 10

Home care advice:

Client comments:

Indemnity: I confirm to the best of my knowledge that I have not withheld any information relevant to my treatment. I understand and accept full responsibility for the treatment that I am given. I also agree that I have given the correct information as detailed on this form and should inform the therapist should these circumstances change.

Client's signature: _____

Therapist's signature: _____   Date: _____

From S. Findlay, 2010, *Sports massage* (Champaign, IL: Human Kinetics).

Closing Remarks

The main purpose of the assessment process is to determine the areas that need intervention, to formulate a plan and to prioritise your goals in a meaningful manner. Your goals will need to be simple, achievable and based on what your client wants. Refrain from pushing forward with a game plan that does not have the agreement of your client despite how much you might believe it is the best thing for them. This approach usually fails. Throughout the process of rehabilitative or corrective work, you will need to revisit some of the tests to assess your client's progress. At the start of any session, approach your client as if it were a first session. Stay alert to any changes or adverse reactions. As any experienced professional will tell you, things do not always go according to plan, so it is important to regularly revisit the assessment process with the aim of being responsive to a client's changing needs.

Quick Questions

1. What is the difference between subjective and objective assessment?
2. What is the difference between intrinsic and extrinsic factors that affect injury?
3. Where on the body should the plumb line run through?
4. During an active test, is the client or the therapist performing the movement?
5. What are eight guidelines for setting effective goals?

10

Event Massage

Event work can be rewarding and challenging and has an air of excitement. The downside can include poor working conditions with low or non-existent monetary rewards and working long hours non-stop. On the flip side, it challenges your ability to respond quickly to a multitude of situations, it develops your skills in a real life situation and is a great opportunity to be able to put your knowledge to work.

CLIENT TALK

Event work can be very inspiring. I remember working at the London Marathon and watching the faces of all those coming down Birdcage Walk Lane to the finish line; the pure determination and emotion that was evident on every face was a moment I would never forget. I then spent the next 5 hours massaging those who had finished. Some were veterans and had done many races and others were first timers, but all had a story to tell that made me realize how special moments like this were, and I was glad I was part of that moment.

Pre-event, post-event and inter-event massage for the most part have different goals and outcomes. The choice of techniques varies, as well as the length of the sessions. Because each type of event work has a purpose and value, you need to be thoughtful and apply the appropriate techniques at the appropriate times.

Pre-Event Massage

Pre-event massage can take place anywhere from a few days to a few minutes before the event. Because its primary purpose is to help prepare the athlete to perform a specific task, it is usually focused on specific muscles. Understanding the demands of the sport will help you decide which muscles to target and the appropriate approach to take to meet the athlete's needs.

Is Pre-Event Massage Appropriate?

To determine whether a pre-event massage is appropriate, consider the following:

- Does the event allow for the application of lubricants?
- What type of event is it? Do you understand the demands of the sport so you can target the muscles that are important for the event?
- Does the athlete need to have quick response times, or is there an element of calmness needed in order to perform his task? Different strokes will create different soft tissue responses (e.g., if they need to be calm use slower strokes, etc).

If an athlete has not had massage before, this is not an appropriate time to start because there is no way of knowing whether massage will adversely affect his performance. Encourage him to have regular maintenance massages between competitions in the future.

What Are the Functions of a Pre-Event Massage?

Pre-event massage has the following functions:

- Optimises performance
- Warms up and increases blood supply to the muscles
- Decreases muscle tension
- Encourages an appropriate range of motion in the joints
- Creates a state of readiness in the muscles
- Allows for mental preparation

When Can Pre-Event Massage Take Place?

Pre-event massage can take place shortly before an event or up to a couple of days before. The closer it is to the event, the more it can be used to enhance an athlete's warm-up; however, it should not replace it. A couple of days before the event, the intention of a massage is less definite. Typically, the purpose will be to give a light flush or stretch to the appropriate areas. You may do some minor treatment but not enough to affect their performance. Generally, pre-event massage is performed within a couple of hours before the event. The duration of the massage is 15 to 20 minutes.

Which Techniques Are Appropriate?

The following techniques can be performed with or without lubrication, working through a towel or directly on the skin depending of the type of sport or the purpose of the massage. The speed or depth at which you apply these techniques will either enhance their performance or could adversely affect it. Be mindful of what the athlete needs. For example, does the athlete need to be calm? If so, use slower, more methodical movements. Alternatively, do they need to be hyped up? Then speed up your work, but always be careful as to how much stress you are placing on the tissue, remembering that the intention is to warm up the tissue rather than perform a treatment. If you use oils or lotions, be sure to wipe them off at the end of the session.

- Effleurage
- Petrissage
- Compression
- Vibration

- Tapotement
- Light friction
- Passive mobility

You might have to be very creative with pre-event massage: you could find yourself working with clients in a standing or seated position rather than having the luxury of a couch at hand. Because clients may not have a place or the time to undress, you might have to work through their kit using dry massage techniques.

Pre-Event Interview Questions

Even in an event setting, it is important to ask questions before beginning a massage. The answers to these questions will help you determine what massage techniques to use and what areas to address.

- How long is it before your event?
- Where are you in your preparation time?
- Are you being treated for any conditions at the present?
- Do you have any conditions at present that will affect your performance?
- Are there any previous injuries that are affecting you today?
- What areas would you like me to work on?
- Is there anything specific you would like me to do?
- Are there any areas of tension that you would like me to focus on or stretch?

Other considerations include an awareness of the potential effect your words can have on the mental state of the athlete. Be careful about what you say; your words can either encourage and relax an athlete or have the opposite effect, which is obviously not your intention. If you believe there is a potential for injury, for example, consult with the appropriate medical or health care professional or the team coach before saying anything to the athlete.

Inter-Event Massage

Inter-event massage combines some of the elements of both the pre- and post-event work. It serves as both preparation for the next event and an evaluation.

Is Inter-Event Massage Appropriate?

The purpose of an inter-event massage is to prepare for the next event as well as to assess for any injuries. It is not a complete recovery massage, but it should help to flush out and prepare the tissue for further work. Because you want to maintain the energy in the muscles and avoid overworking and weakening them, consider the speed and depth of your application.

What Are the Functions of an Inter-Event Massage?

Inter-event massage has the following functions:

- Improves recovery
- Prepares the athlete for the next event
- Delivers a focused and specific massage

When Can Inter-Event Massage Take Place?

Inter-event massage is performed between events taking place on the same day, such as at halftime or between heats. The duration is between 5 and 10 minutes.

Which Techniques Are Appropriate?

Because you will not have an abundance of time to deliver an inter-event massage, you must know the sport so you can deliver an efficient, effective and targeted massage. Athletes will often direct you to the areas that they would like you to focus on. You may only need to address a small area of tissue tension or restriction and apply a few basic techniques rather than a full massage sequence. The pace of delivery is faster than that of a normal massage, but it should not be too fast or too slow; the intention is to help the client recover and prepare for the next performance, not to sedate him.

The following techniques are appropriate for an inter-event massage:

- Effleurage
- Petrissage
- Compression
- Vibration
- Tapotement
- Light friction
- Mobility

Inter-Event Interview Questions

Even in an event setting, it is important to ask questions before beginning a massage. The answers to the following questions will help you determine what massage techniques to use and what areas to address.

- How long is it before your event?
- Are you being treated for any conditions at the present?
- Did you have any problems during the event?
- Are there any specific areas you would like me to work on?
- Are there any areas of tension that you would like me to focus on?

Post-Event Massage

Post-event massage is the most common form of event massage, and volunteer situations are often plentiful. Volunteering is a great way to be introduced to the art of event work and learn about the requirements of each sport. Frequently, you will get someone new to massage after an event such as a marathon, which can be an opportunity to educate the person about the benefits of regular massage.

Is Post-Event Massage Appropriate?

The main purposes of post-event massage is to bring the tissues back to a pre-event state by flushing them out, and to be observant and identify any injuries or conditions that need first aid or further medical attention. If a medical team is not doing post-event assessments, you will need to do a consultation prior to starting the massage. You must be aware of the signs and symptoms of the most common problems and be equipped to deal with them.

What Are the Functions of a Post-Event Massage?

Post-event massage has the following functions:

- Assesses for injuries or tissue damage
- Normalises tissue
- Restores muscle tone
- Restores resting muscle length
- Flushes out any congested areas
- Prevents muscle soreness
- Restores flexibility
- Relieves muscle cramps and spasms
- Supports metabolic recovery

When Can Post-Event Massage Take Place?

Ideally, post-event massage should take place within 2 to 6 hours after the event. This is the most effective time in which to work, but massage can still be very beneficial after a couple of days. The duration of the massage should be 15 to 20 minutes. The greater the time since the event, the longer the massage can be.

Which Techniques Are Appropriate?

The following techniques can be used during post-event massage sessions:

- Effleurage
- Petrissage
- Gentle compression
- Stretching
- General massage application
- Superficial depth
- Lymphatic drainage

Post-Event Interview Questions

Even in an event setting, it is important to ask questions before beginning a massage. The answers to these questions will help you determine what massage techniques to use and what areas to address.

- Have you completed your post-event cool-down?
- Did you have any problems during the event?
- Can you identify any areas of pain or soreness?
- Are you feeling hot, warm or cold?
- Have you had a post-event hydration drink or snack?
- Are you suffering from dizziness, headaches, confusion, unsteadiness or nausea?

In addition to asking these questions, you need to be aware of the following common post-event conditions, because they will influence the treatment you give.

- Blisters
- Contusions
- Cramps
- Dehydration or over hydration
- Heat exhaustion

- Hyperthermia
- Hypothermia
- Open wounds
- Sprains
- Strains

If you are qualified to give first aid and the injuries are minor, you can treat as appropriate. When in doubt, refer the person to a qualified professional. If a health team is available, typically they are at the forefront, screening clients and taking care of first aid situations. However, if you are the only one available, you will be expected to have the appropriate training to assess for conditions that would warrant medical treatment. Those with serious conditions should always be sent to a medical facility.

Working With an Elite Sport Team

Working with an elite sport team and being part of the team's success is a wholly rewarding experience, but it has to be remembered that there are no 'Olympic Games for massage therapists'. Our role is about supporting the athletes and helping them along the journey to their own ultimate success!

Working within a performance medical team is totally different from working autonomously in a clinic environment. Having the skill of autonomy is indeed a part of it, but the accountability and responsibility of the support staff must not be taken light-heartedly. Each person within the medical team should have a defined role with clear parameters for each of those roles, coupled with an obvious hierarchy to ensure ultimate responsibility. Each member of the medical team needs to be able to understand the roles of all the other members and how these roles overlap and compliment each other once the competition has started. This not only ensures the athletes are provided with what they require but also makes sure the work load is spread throughout the team; performance environments can be very stressful! As a sports massage therapist or soft tissue therapist (as the role is titled in performance sport now), the role is ultimately to support the work of a physiotherapist and the other medical professionals within the team, but it is primarily to 'do exactly as it says on the tin'. Your role within a high performance team is to look after the athletes' soft tissues primarily–muscles!

Massage is a very useful and powerful medium that can help in all aspects of preparation and recovery. Anecdotally, there is also something inherent in the physical nature of touch. It lets the athletes know that they are in safe hands and that there is the support for all the efforts that they are required to put forth, both for able-bodied athletes and athletes with disabilities. One of the key things to remember when working with athletes with disabilities is that first and foremost, they are athletes! Yes, in some instances disabled athletes may require greater amounts of support to facilitate their own success, but the work is in effect the same. (For more information on working with special populations, see chapter 11.)

As the athletes have spent a long time preparing for competition, it is imperative that you are also prepared for the demands that are ahead of you. It is useful to plan the logistics that will be required for the days of competition, from identifying where you will be treating the team to the transportation that will be available to and from the competition venue, as this can easily add to the physical workload if you have to carry a couch on and off the transport and walk it up and down flights of stairs and in and out of venues.

Then there are the athletes. You need to understand what each athlete's particular objectives are during the competition; when will they require help in preparing for races, what will they require as recovery and is there any specific intervention that is required as part of an injury management strategy? Understanding each of the athletes' requirements will help you plan the days, ensure everyone gets what they require and make sure that you are prepared for the demands of the day. This can be a tough call if you are travelling with a large team. It takes time to case conference individual's needs and this often has to be done at the beginning or end of the day. During the Paralympic Games held in Beijing in 2008, the medical team's day started at 5:15 am and finished around 10:30 pm for the nine consecutive days of competition. It was quite exhausting!

What is absolutely necessary is to prepare yourself physically for the competition. The days can be very long and can be very intense no matter what level of competition. Whether the Olympic Games or domestic trials, all competitions are strenuous. Making sure you have the strength and fitness to work multiple days in a row with lots of hours of massage every day is vitally important. It is no good for the team to break down without anyone to look after the important people: the athletes!

With the obvious physical demands of continuous massage on a daily basis, the psychological impact of the environment also can be very challenging. Tensions run very high and emotions can swing between the extremes in an instant. This can be very draining to those immersed in the competition. A useful part to the end of day debrief is to debrief yourself. Talking through the day's events with the rest of the support staff is a necessary and valuable experience.

In all, working within a performance team environment is a unique and incredible experience, but it is the preparation for the inevitable demands that is essential to ensure that it is everything that you would ever want it to be–one of the most memorable and rewarding experiences of your life.

The above section was contributed by Elizabeth Soames, Working Bodies Fitness & Injury Centre, Towcester, Northamptonshire, England. Elizabeth provides soft tissue massage therapy to Badminton England, Disability Swimming, English Institute of Sport, England Ladies Cricket and Hertfordshire County Cricket. She is the association director of Working Bodies Ltd.

Organising an Event

Organising any event can be very demanding regardless of the size. It requires good organisational and communication skills and, at times, a great deal of diplomacy. It does not usually have a large monetary value attached to it, but it is an experience that does offer opportunities to develop as a therapist and to make connections with colleagues. Organising an event can give you an opportunity to promote your services, especially if you work at events close to your own turf.

Event size ranges from major events to smaller ones at local clubs. At the beginning of your career, or during your studies, start by volunteering at a few supervised events to get the necessary experience before venturing out on your own.

First Steps

Approach your local club or a charity and offer your services. If there is an event organiser, contact that person to make sure there is a need for your services and to find out whether someone else has already been hired for the job. Clearly define your scope of responsibility. Are you working with other team members? If so, who are they (i.e., physiotherapist, doctor, etc)? You will need to know how many participants there are in order to determine if you are working on your own or if there is a need for more therapists, which might require you to take on a more supervisory role. Also find out whether there are any protocols for your type of service (e.g., you might not be allowed to charge if it is a charitable event, or there may be restrictions about where you can work). It is important to get letters of agreement in writing and supply any necessary documents such as copies of insurance or the qualifications of therapists you will be providing. Make sure to do the following:

- Determine the size of the event and the number of participants and how many massage sessions will be provided.
- Establish the protocol for referring to the medical team.
- Find out who will provide and pay for supplies, transportation and parking.
- Decide whether to offer freebies such a T-shirts to massage volunteers.
- Decide whether to provide water and food.
- Arrange parking, kit storage and any other concerns.
- Determine security measures. (Will therapists need identification badges to get into the event?)

Book your therapists in advance including a few extras. People do cancel, and quite often at the last hour. It is better to have too many (this way everyone can get breaks) than too few. Having too few therapists can lead to your team being overworked and not enjoying the event experience. Also, participants can end up being turned away and will share their disgruntlement with the organisers, which might result in your not being asked back again for future events.

Remember to thank the organiser and any volunteers for their part of the day.

Organising the Venue

Event organisers might expect you to provide your own tent or might not have a suitable place for you to work, so be prepared and assess the situation beforehand. Even in the summer it is advisable to have a covered area in which to work for your own comfort as well as that of the participants. Make sure you are not stuck in a corner where no one can see or find you; you should be central to the activity so people know you are there. Work out in advance how you are going to get to the venue, how long it will take to get there and whether there is any place to store equipment. Setting up the day before is ideal. Make sure you also do the following:

- Arrange couches to accommodate the flow of people.
- Set up an area where people can register, sign release forms and wait for their sessions.
- If a medical team is doing post-event assessments to determine whether people are fit for massages, allow time for this.
- Set up a rota for breaks, possibly sharing the supervisory or management role.
- Put up any signage or banners.
- If you have any personal business cards, be sure to have them handy.

Supplies and Equipment Checklist

Be sure you are prepared for the event! If after all your advanced planning, you have forgotten equipment or supplies, it can take away from the success of the event. Following is a checklist of supplies and equipment to have on hand:

TIP Dress appropriately, including layers of clothing to accommodate hot and cold conditions. Remember to bring sunscreen because you may end up working out in the open without any protection.

- Treatment couch (if not supplied)
- Pillows or cushions
- Towels (large and small)
- Couch roll
- Antiseptic wipes
- Massage lotion
- Bin liners to put used couch rolls in, etc.
- First aid kit (pins, scissors, adhesive tape, gauze, cold packs, sugary product)
- Clock to keep an eye on treatment times (a nurse's watch is very useful)
- Business cards or any advertising you have put together
- Camera to take photos for memorabilia or future advertising
- Water and snacks for yourself
- Fully charged mobile phone, but have it on vibration
- Stationery to organise client lists (tickets for bookings)
- Pens
- A cash float if you are charging for treatments

Closing Remarks

Students and graduates alike find the experience of working at events helpful for developing their skills and understanding the demands of sport. They find this kind of work hard but exhilarating. The type of event can range from working as a team member on a long-haul trip to volunteering for a day at a charity event such as a marathon. These are exciting moments and should be a part of every sports massage therapist's training.

Quick Questions

1. What are the primary differences between pre- and post-event massage?
2. Which soft tissue techniques are appropriate for post-event massage?
3. What are the three primary reasons for performing intra-event massage?
4. Which one of the following is *not* a common condition found in a post-event situation?

Blisters	Diarrhoea
Contusions	Heat exhaustion
Cramps	Hypothermia
Dehydration or overhydration	Sprains

5. If someone is new to massage, should you massage him for the first time prior to an event?

Special Populations

For the purpose of this book, special populations include clients with specific conditions that require a greater understanding of their physiology and soft tissue issues (e.g., a Paralympic athlete). At the elite level, athletes with disabilities are categorised as having either a physical disability or intellectual impairment. To permit fair competition, people with physical disabilities are categorised as follows:

- Spinal cord injury (congenital or acquired)
- Limb deficiency or amputation and les autres (from the French meaning 'the others')—physical disabilities such as muscular dystrophies, restricted growth, syndromic conditions and ankylosis or arthritis of major joints that do not fit within the other categories
- Cerebral palsy
- Visual impairment (blind or partially sighted)

Athletes with these conditions may need help getting on and off the couch. You will also have to consider which techniques would be suitable and which you should avoid. In addition to understanding how to physically manage clients with these conditions, you need to understand the physiological effects of their conditions. They might have a loss of sensation, or they might suffer with poor tissue health that slows their ability to heal. The better you understand their condition, their needs and how to make appropriate adjustments, the more effective the massage will be.

Spinal Cord Injuries

Spinal cord injuries can be a result of a disease such as polio or spina bifida, but they are more commonly a result of trauma such as falls and motor vehicle accidents. The management of spinal cord injuries is dictated by the degree of paralysis and function. This depends on the location of the injury on the spinal cord. Quadriplegia and tetraplegia result from injuries to the cervical region (neck); paraplegia involves the thoracic, lumbar or sacral area. The higher the location of the lesion, the greater the loss of body function.

Transferring

The first thing to do with a client who has a spinal cord injury is to ask if he needs any help transferring to the couch. Many choose to transfer themselves, directing the therapist to help as needed. Also, do not assume that an athlete in a wheelchair cannot walk.

If you have a couch that cannot be adjusted easily to accommodate a person with a spinal cord injury, an alternative is to massage the person in the wheelchair. Before beginning, make sure the brakes are on. Position the wheelchair so the person can lean forward onto the couch, using pillows to support her as necessary. This will allow you to access most of the trunk, working from the side or from behind.

Position Management

Managing and supporting the limbs of a client with no motor control requires a greater awareness on your part. For instance, when moving a client from a prone to a side-lying position, you will have to support and control the legs. If the legs are allowed to drop unrestrained, the impact and force from the movement can cause tissue and structural damage. Lack of motor control may also cause muscular spasms when the person is moving into certain positions (e.g. from prone to supine), so be prepared for unexpected movements or shaking. Even though there is a loss of sensory perception, maintain your protocols for limb support (e.g., place cushions under the knees).

Sensation

In addition to a loss of function, a person with a spinal cord injury can have an altered perception of sensation and may not be able to feel pain or a light touch. Therefore, you will need to adjust the depth and speed of your stroke, starting off lighter and slower until you are familiar with the client's tolerance levels. Remember also that any tissue that cannot reflexively contract cannot protect itself and will be vulnerable to damage. Therefore, it is important to adjust your monitoring and evaluation techniques based on your client's situation.

Thermoregulation

People with spinal cord injuries have an autonomic dysfunction that alters thermo-regulation, impairing their ability to control their body temperature below the level of the injury. They lack the ability to respond to cold and cannot shiver to stay warm. As a result, they might require more towels to maintain a comfortable degree of warmth. At the other end of the spectrum, they are also vulnerable to heat illness because the cooling mechanism is also impaired. Be aware of the signs and symptoms of heat stroke, hyperthermia and heat exhaustion so that you will know when it is appropriate to refer a patient. (See the Pathology section in chapter 2.)

People with spinal cord injuries are also susceptible to a condition called hyper-reflexia, or autonomic dysreflexia, which is an excessive response of the involuntary nervous system (autonomic) as a result of nerve impulses triggered by normal stimuli; for example, when the bladder is full and the signal does not reach the brain. This excessive response can also be caused by intestinal blockages and by physical constriction (e.g., if the athlete competes with strapping to hold her in position). This extreme reaction can cause a change in the heart rate, increased blood pressure, changes in skin colour and excessive sweating. Hyperreflexia is considered a medical emergency and needs immediate attention.

Osteopenia

As a consequence of immobility, the athlete can suffer from a condition called osteopenia, which is a decrease in bone mineral density. This thinning of the bones increases the risk of fractures (osteoporosis). In such cases, you will need to modify your technique and method of application. Avoid any heavy-handed tapotement or vibrations or any excessive pressure to the affected areas. Because the person may also lack any sensation of pain or discomfort, it is important to watch for signs of a fracture. This could be evidenced by the bone feeling out of alignment with the rest of the bone, any abnormal movement or if there is any evidence of bruising or bleeding. In the last case, refer the person to the medical team.

Massage Considerations

Wheelchair users, or those who have to use their shoulders and arms to transfer themselves from place to place, are prone to shoulder overuse injuries. It is common to have repetitive strain issues, scoliosis due to poor seating position and muscle imbalances that result from pushing techniques. These may all contribute to alterations in scapula stabilisation and abnormal patterns of movement. The aim of the massage session would be to address these issues and work within a team setting (which could include a doctor, physio, coach, trainer, etc.) to make the corrective adjustments. Remember that some stiffness may be functional (e.g., erector spinae to maintain an upright posture) and is therefore desirable.

Often, the areas we concentrate on are those that are being used, but the benefits of massage are global. Flushing techniques can enhance tissue quality especially in the areas that are incapable of maintaining a natural pumping action. Regular massage may also reduce the frequency of muscle spasms.

Areas of contact are also susceptible to skin abrasions or pressure sores from prolonged sitting and poor tissue quality. The key is prevention and increasing circulation to the area, as well as movement. Regular inspection of these areas is an important feature in prevention.

Finally, as a result of altered geometry and a decrease in the use of their limbs, people with spinal cord injuries can be predisposed to developing joint contractures. By lengthening and stretching the soft tissue, you can help maintain the integrity of the joint and its adjoining structures.

Limb Deficiency

Limb deficiencies may be congenital or acquired. Athletes with limb deficiencies compete with or without prostheses or in wheelchairs. Prostheses can be worn on the upper and lower extremities. Both can affect functional movement patterns causing postural imbalances. For instance, because a prosthetic lower limb is shorter than the unaffected limb (to allow the person to swing the leg through), a muscle imbalance can develop from the altered gait, which may cause pelvic or low back pain. Prostheses can also cause skin chafing, abrasion and bone bruising.

Massage considerations include addressing muscle imbalances by lengthening or stretching tight muscles followed by strengthening weaker ones. Local contraindications include sores, swelling and a mangled or infected stump. Prostheses are usually removed before a massage; sometimes the stump is covered with a soft cover. Generally the stump can be massaged like any other area of the body, unless inflammation or abrasions are present. Always ask permission to massage a stump. Some athletes may be very sensitive to having it worked on. Others may not be used to having someone other than their doctors touch it.

Cerebral Palsy

Cerebral palsy is characterised by a variety of movement disorders that are classified by how many limbs are affected and the symptoms they produce. The primary characteristics are a large amount of involuntary movement, poor coordination, and hyper- or hypotonia. Others might include epilepsy, deafness, learning impairment and visual and speech defects; these can also occur in combination. Cerebral palsy can be classified as follows:

- Monoplegia—One limb is affected, usually an arm.
- Paraplegia—The lower extremities and hip region are affected.
- Hemiplegia—Limbs on one side of the body are affected.
- Triplegia—Three limbs are affected, usually both legs and one arm.
- Quadriplegia—All four limbs and the trunk are affected. Neck and facial muscles may also be involved.
- Diplegia—More involvement in the lower limbs than in the upper limbs.

Broadly speaking, those that live with cerebral palsy have difficulty with muscle tone and cannot contract or relax certain muscles. As the bones grow, the muscles and tendons can remain shortened, which can lead to pain. A number of options are available to alleviate or minimise the effects of the condition—having surgery, taking medication to relax the overactive tissue and wearing braces on the legs and arms to stretch the muscles and tendons. A classic pattern of muscle contraction results in flexion, adduction and internal rotation. The overall aim of a sports massage is to improve posture and mobility and reduce muscle contractures.

For athletes who suffer with a spastic form of cerebral palsy, ensure their safety by offering the appropriate amount of physical support, but do not restrict their movements. Rather, maintain an appropriate level of guidance and cushioning.

Visual Impairment

There are three levels of classifications for visual impairment as defined by Parasport (www.uka.org.uk):

B1 (blind)—Unable to recognise the form of a hand in any direction or at any distance.

B2 (partially sighted)—Able to recognise the shape of a hand to a visual acuity of 2/60 and/or a visual field of less than 5 degrees.

B3 (visually impaired)—Has a visual acuity of greater than 2/60 up to 6/60 and/or a visual field of greater than 5 degrees and less than 20 degrees.

Make sure your massage room is clear of any unwanted articles on the floor or wires that clients could trip over. If a client with a visual impairment is not familiar with the surroundings and needs assistance, gently take her arm in a supported manner or allow her to hold your arm at the elbow and physically guide her to the couch or chair giving verbal directions at the same time. Guide the person carefully around any sharp corners on couches or other furniture. (This is one of the reasons to purchase a padded couch with rounded corners.)

Having continuity within your massage is an important skill. Alerting your client about your intentions will create trust and relaxation. If you finish with one part of the body and move to another without communicating this through hand or verbal cues, the client may find your actions unpredictable and feel invaded. Be clear about your intentions and remain in contact as much as possible.

Communication

In all of the aforementioned conditions, good communication skills are vital. Be an active listener and take extra care in repeating back to the client any information she has given you. If a client suffers with a speech defect, as is the case with some forms of cerebral palsy, be patient and give her time to communicate. It is important that you have a comprehensive understanding of her symptoms as well as a full history because this will affect the success of your treatment. If an athlete has difficulty hearing, make sure she can see your face when you speak. There is no need to speak louder or exaggerate your words; the client should understand if you speak in a thoughtful manner. Giving clear instructions will not only help to ensure the safety of your client when moving her on and off the couch, but can increase the effectiveness of your treatment when client participation is necessary.

Closing Remarks

Working with clients that have special needs requires sensitivity and insight in order to accommodate their functional limitations; focus on the ability and not the disability. You will need to modify your techniques, have excellent communication skills and be able to use your imagination when faced with unusual requirements. Experience is often your best teacher that will help develop these skills, as well as getting to know each individual's specific needs. It takes time, patience and a good sense of humor (on both sides).

Quick Questions

1. When a client with a spinal cord injury is moving into certain positions, what can a lack of motor control cause?
2. What must you be sure to do with a wheelchair to ensure a client's safety before moving your client onto the couch?
3. What is an effect of the altered gait that results from wearing a prosthesis?
4. What part of the body does paraplegia affect?
5. How should you prepare a room for someone who is visually impaired?

Answers to Quick Questions

Chapter 1

1. Sports massage is not exclusive to those engaged in sport, but is for anyone who has an interest in soft tissue work and feels she can benefit from this form of massage.

2. Sports massage can release soft tissue tension, relieve stiffness, decrease muscle spasms, release restrictions, soften and realign scar tissue and loosen up adhesions, helping to restore optimal function.

3. Any time a client desires soft tissue massage.

4. To assist the athlete to achieve peak performance and remain injury free as well as to support the healing process of any injuries.

5. Sports massage therapists should be able to perform an appropriate range of assessment and evaluation processes, as well as recognise common sports injuries. They should also be able to design and implement comprehensive treatment plans with realistic and achievable goals.

Chapter 2

1. *Global* means that the massage is contraindicated altogether because the condition affects the body systemically, whereas *local* means that massage can take place but away from the area of consideration.

2. *Severe, acute, uncontrolled, undiagnosed* and *contagious*. Other conditions do not contain these words but are considered contraindications. Be aware of this when deciding whether to continue. If you are unsure, do not proceed.

3. Modifications needed include the choice of technique; whether to work specifically or generally, or superficially or deeply; the direction and speed of the movement; the duration of the massage; the stage of tissue healing; and the positioning of the client.

4. *Global:* Flu and colds, severe pain; *Local:* acute scar tissue, open wounds, folliculitis; *Modification:* Whiplash, diabetes, cancer, old dislocation of the shoulder, osteoporosis.

5. A sprain involves ligaments and the joint, whereas a strain involves soft tissue such as muscle and tendons.

Chapter 3

1. Working alongside other professionals, receiving support from other team members, having a receptionist handle your appointments, having a couch and towels supplied.
2. Direct contact, indirect contact, and air transmission.
3. Comfort, stability, joint and limb support.
4. Ankles, hip, torso, and shoulders.
5. It allows the body to rest in a more natural position, giving ease to the lower back, while preventing the knee joint from being forced beyond a normal range of motion.

Chapter 4

1.
   - Keep your hips and shoulders squared.
   - Adopt a wide stance.
   - Place your arms away from your body.
   - Maintain long levers.
   - Create a circle with your arms.
   - Do not lock your elbows.
   - Generate movement from your legs.
2. Reassess your application technique, take care of yourself by keeping fit, stretch and have a regular massage.
3. Go slower.
4. Muscle tension, clenching of fists, twitching elsewhere in the body, a pushing out action of the muscle being worked on, red ears, all-over body perspiration, verbal response.
5. The legs.

Chapter 5

1. To warm up the tissue, to prepare it for deeper work and to assess it for areas of tension or areas that need further attention.
2. Effleurage, compression, vibration, light tapotement.
3. Fragile skin, neighbouring infections, recent scar tissue and decreased sensation (i.e., diabetes).
4. The physiological conditions of the client, sensitive structures and bony prominences.
5. Slower.

Chapter 6

1. A seated position on the couch allows you to access areas anterior to the shoulder that are restrictive in nature. It can also help to prepare the area for more specific work before moving the client into another position.

2. A lot!

3. That there is nothing with regards to your clothing that will cause discomfort and that you maintain professional modesty by placing a towel between yourself and your client.

4. Because the surface area of the foot is small and the depth of the tissue is nominal, working with the thumbs and digits is not stressful. The foot also requires a more precise application of techniques because of the small working area.

5. The neck.

Chapter 7

1. Once you have mastered the basic working massage positions.

2. Under the head and knees.

3. Clockwise.

4. Direct your gaze away from the area, work through a towel and work confidently.

5. The feet play an integral role in the movement and function of the whole body.

Chapter 8

1. Under the head and top bent leg. You may also place one under the torso above the hips to open up the space between the ribs and hip.

2. The height of the client's hip is significantly higher in a side-lying position than it is in a prone or a supine position.

3. When you want to access soft tissue using an alternative method, since it allows for the muscle to drop away from the skeletal structure. You can get underneath or behind an area rather than having to press through other more superficial tissue.

4. To stabilise the client's position and to keep her hips and back in alignment.

5. You can ask her to hold the couch with her free hand, bending her arm at a 90-degree angle.

Chapter 9

1. Subjective assessment is the stage in which you take a client's history, including a medical history and information about the client's training regime and typical

activities. During the objective assessment stage you do physical assessments using palpation and postural, ROM and functional tests.

2. Intrinsic factors are internal conditions that influence injury (e.g., past injuries), whereas extrinsic factors are those that come from outside (i.e., the environment).

3. ▪ Slightly anterior to the ankle
   ▪ Slightly anterior to the centre of the knee
   ▪ Just posterior to the centre of the hip joint
   ▪ Through the centre of the shoulder joint
   ▪ Through the ear lobe

4. The client is performing the movement.

5. ▪ Set goals that are challenging and realistic
   ▪ Set goals that are specific, based on behaviour and measurable
   ▪ Set both process and outcome goals
   ▪ Use positive terminology
   ▪ Establish a comprehensive timetable for goal completion
   ▪ Monitor and evaluate progress
   ▪ Focus on degrees of achievement
   ▪ Make goals personal

Chapter 10

1. Pre-event massage is for preparing the tissue to perform a task, whereas post-event massage is about restoring the tissue to its pre-event condition.

2. Effleurage
   Petrissage
   Gentle compression
   Stretching
   General massage application
   Superficial depth
   Lymphatic drainage

3. To improve recovery
   To prepare for the next event
   To deliver a focused and specific massage

4. Diarrhoea.

5. It is generally inappropriate primarily because you do not know how he will react to the massage, whether it will have an adverse affect or whether his system can cope.

Chapter 11

1. Muscle spasms.
2. Put on the brakes.
3. Muscle imbalance.
4. The lower extremities and hip region.
5. Make sure the room is clear of any unwanted articles on the floor or wires that the person could trip over.

PRONE

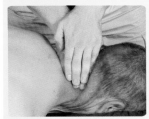

Neck
p. 69

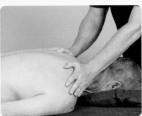

Shoulder
p. 70

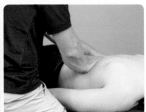

Torso
p. 74

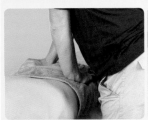

Pelvis
p. 76

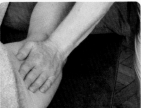

Legs
p. 78

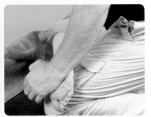

Feet
p. 82

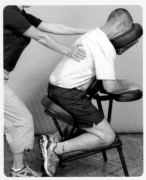

Sitting
p. 83

SUPINE

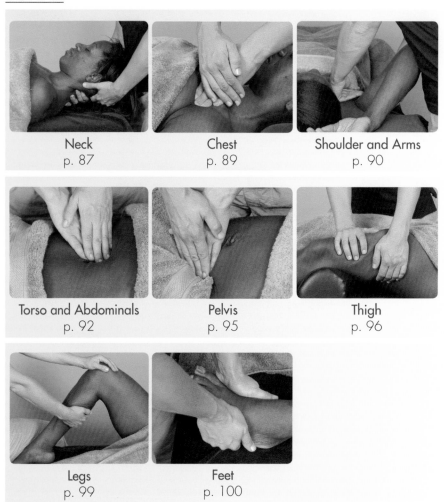

Neck
p. 87

Chest
p. 89

Shoulder and Arms
p. 90

Torso and Abdominals
p. 92

Pelvis
p. 95

Thigh
p. 96

Legs
p. 99

Feet
p. 100

SIDE-LYING

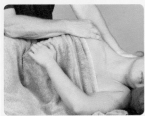

Neck
p. 103

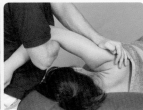

Shoulders and Arms
p. 105

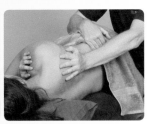

Torso
p. 107

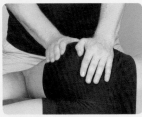

Pelvis
p. 109

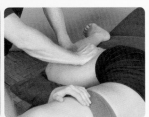

Thigh
p. 110

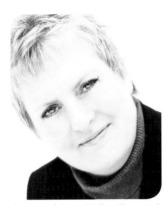

Courtesy of Susan Findlay. Photograph by Jo de Banzie.

Susan Findlay, BSc RGN, Dip SRMT, is director of the North London School of Sports Massage, where she is a sport and remedial massage therapist and lecturer. Findlay's experiences as a ballet dancer, gymnast, personal trainer, and nurse have allowed her to develop both an applied and a clinical understanding of human movement, physical activity, anatomy, and physiology. Findlay is the co-founder of the Institute of Sport and Remedial Massage. She also serves as chair of communications on the General Council of Massage Therapy and as an educational advisor to the Sport Massage Association. In her free time, Findlay enjoys motorbiking, cycling, and yoga.

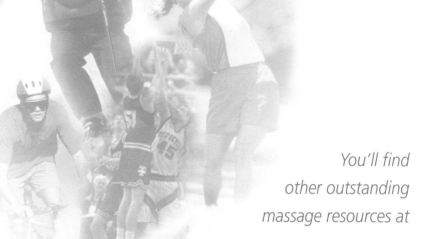

*You'll find
other outstanding
massage resources at*

www.HumanKinetics.com

United States	1-800-747-4457
Australia	08 8372 0999
Canada	1-800-465-7301
Europe	+44 (0) 113 255 5665
New Zealand	0800 222 062

 HUMAN KINETICS
The Information Leader in Physical Activity & Health
P.O. Box 5076 • Champaign, IL 61825-5076 USA